Ureteral Stone Management

Sutchin R. Patel • Stephen Y. Nakada
Editors

Ureteral Stone Management

A Practical Approach

Springer

Editors
Sutchin R. Patel
Department of Urology
University of Wisconsin School
of Medicine and Public Health
Madison, WI
USA

Stephen Y. Nakada
Department of Urology
University of Wisconsin School
of Medicine and Public Health
Madison, WI
USA

ISBN 978-3-319-08791-7 ISBN 978-3-319-08792-4 (eBook)
DOI 10.1007/978-3-319-08792-4
Springer Cham Heidelberg New York Dordrecht London

Library of Congress Control Number: 2014956016

Printed on acid-free paper

Springer is part of Springer Science+Business Media (www.springer.com)

I would like to thank my family for their support in all of my endeavors (my parents, grandparents, Geena and Farina), my mentors in Urology – who have taught me so much and whom I model my practice on (Dr. Stephen Nakada, Dr. Gyan Pareek, Dr. Anthony Caldamone and Dr. Mark Sigman) – and the many chapter authors for their hard work and without whom this text would not be possible.

This text is dedicated to Dr. August Zabbo (1953–2007), who first introduced me to endourology and who taught me that success in the field "requires patience and sometimes being more stubborn than the stone."

Sutchin R. Patel

Contents

Contributors

Sara L. Best, MD Department of Urology, University of Wisconsin School of Medicine and Public Health, Madison, WI, USA

Ben H. Chew, MD Department of Urologic Sciences, University of British Columbia, Level 6 - 2775 Laurel St., Vancouver, BC, V5Z 1M9, Canada

Jonathan Cloutier Department of Urology, Tenon Hospital, Pierre et Marie Curie University, Paris, France

Sarah L. Coleman Department of Endourology and Stone Disease, Stevan Streem Center, Cleveland Clinic Foundation, Cleveland, OH, USA

Mordechai Duvdevani Department of Urology, Hadassah Ein-Kerem University Hospital, The Hebrew University, Jerusalem, Israel

Sammy Elsamra The Smith Institute for Urology, Hofstra North Shore Long Island Jewish School of Medicine, New Hyde Park, NY, USA

Samuel Haywood, MD Department of Urology, The Cleveland Clinic, Cleveland, OH, USA

David Hoenig The Smith Institute for Urology, Hofstra North Shore Long Island Jewish School of Medicine, New Hyde Park, NY, USA

Marcel Hruza, MD Department of Urology, SLK Kliniken Heilbronn, University of Heidelberg, Heilbronn, Germany

Amy E. Krambeck, MD Department of Urology, Mayo Clinic, Rochester, MN, USA

Dirk Lange, MD Department of Urologic Sciences, University of British Columbia 2660 Oak St., Vancouver, BC, V6H 3C6, Canada

David Leavitt The Smith Institute for Urology, Hofstra North Shore Long Island Jewish School of Medicine, New Hyde Park, NY, USA

Michael E. Lipkin, MD Division of Urology, Duke University Medical Center, Durham, NC, USA

Michael Maddox Department of Urology, Tulane University School of Medicine, New Orleans, LA, USA

Manoj Monga Department of Endourology and Stone Disease, Stevan Streem Center, Cleveland Clinic Foundation, Cleveland, OH, USA

Michael E. Moran, MD Curator, William P. Didusch Center for Urologic History, Linthicum, MD, USA

Stephen Y. Nakada, MD Department of Urology, University of Wisconsin School of Medicine and Public Health, Madison, WI, USA

Zeph Okeke The Smith Institute for Urology, Hofstra North Shore Long Island Jewish School of Medicine, New Hyde Park, NY, USA

Gyan Pareek, MD Division of Urology, The Warren Alpert Medical School of Brown University, Providence, RI, USA

Sutchin R. Patel, MD Department of Urology, University of Wisconsin School of Medicine and Public Health, Madison, WI, USA

Ryan F. Paterson, MD Department of Urologic Sciences, University of British Columbia, Level 6 - 2775 Laurel St., Vancouver, BC, V5Z 1M9 Canada

Mary Powers Department of Urology, Tulane University School of Medicine, New Orleans, LA, USA

Jens Rassweiler, MD Department of Urology, SLK Kliniken Heilbronn, University of Heidelberg, Heilbronn, Germany

Marcelino E. Rivera, MD Department of Urology, Mayo Clinic, Rochester, MN, USA

Stavros Sfoungaristos Department of Urology, Hadassah Hebrew University Medical Center, Jerusalem, Israel

Sri Sivalingam, MD Department of Urology, The Cleveland Clinic, Cleveland, OH, USA

Necole M. Streeper Department of Urology, University of Wisconsin School of Medicine and Public Health, Madison, WI, USA

Abdulkadir Tepeler Department of Urology, University of Wisconsin School of Medicine and Public Health, Madison, WI, USA

Raju Thomas Department of Urology, Tulane University School of Medicine, New Orleans, LA, USA

Tim Tran, MD Division of Urology, The Warren Alpert Medical School of Brown University, Providence, RI, USA

Olivier Traxer Department of Urology, Tenon Hospital, Pierre et Marie Curie University, Paris, France

Chapter 1
History of the Treatment of Ureteral Calculi

Sutchin R. Patel and Michael E. Moran

Ureteral Stones: A Brief History

Ureteral calculi have been reported prior to the modern era of surgical intervention, but literally nothing could be done for them. There is almost no literature on their incidence or their treatments since there was little that could be done. Three titanic innovations in medicine were necessary for these stones to be able to be treated in the modern era: anesthesia, antiseptic and aseptic surgery and the near synchronous discovery of X-rays. With both a diagnosis and an effective therapeutic alternative in place the stage would now be set for the rapid development of less invasive methods for treatment based upon the foundation stones of modern urology- the cystoscope [1].

One well known historical vignette is in order to begin this chapter. Samuel Pepys, perhaps best known for his bladder stone and surgical intervention, recorded, "*I remember not my life without the pain of the stone in the kidneys* (*even to the making of bloody water upon any extraordinary motion*) *until I was about twenty years of age*" [2]. He would later become a student at Trinity Hall, Cambridge, where he passed a ureteral calculus in the summer of 1653. He described the classic symptoms of ureteral colic which he believed was brought about by a long walk. Mr. Thomas Hollier of St. Thomas Hospital finally cut on Pepys for this stone on March 26, 1658 and this left a lifetime impression on him [3]. Nothing could be done for stones in the upper tracts until some of the most significant advances in medicine and surgery could be developed and even then there were lessons to be learned.

S.R. Patel, MD (✉)
Department of Urology, University of Wisconsin School of Medicine and Public Health, Madison, WI, USA
e-mail: sutchin_patel@yahoo.com

M.E. Moran, MD
Curator, William P. Didusch Center for Urologic History, Linthicum, MD, USA

S.R. Patel, S.Y. Nakada (eds.), *Ureteral Stone Management: A Practical Approach*, DOI 10.1007/978-3-319-08792-4_1

Antiseptic to Aseptic Surgery

As the medical side of stone disease advanced at the dawn of the twentieth century, so too did surgical intervention. Spurred on by some of the greatest developments in the history of medicine itself, some believed that the late nineteenth and early twentieth centuries marked the high-point of surgical science. Let's begin with the founder of aseptic surgery, Baron Joseph Lister (1827–1912). Lister was born on April 5, 1827 to a well off Quaker family and his father was the famous Joseph Jackson Lister who invented the compound microscope and achromatic lenses that aided another brilliant Quaker physician, Thomas Hodgkin's work in pathology [4]. He attended the University of London and graduated with honors as Bachelor of Medicine and entered the Royal College of Surgeons at age 26. He moved to the University of Edinburgh to work with James Syme and eventually married Syme's eldest daughter Agnes who became his chief research assistant. He moved to the University of Glasgow as professor of surgery [5]. He had read Louis Pasteur's work on microbes and investigated the use of carbolic acid to reduce the infection rates of wounds. As a young surgeon he was distressed by his high rate of post operative infections. "Hospitalism" had been coined to describe the widespread belief that being in an institution often was associated with bad outcomes [6]. In August, 1865 he applied carbolic acid soaked dressings to a compound fracture on an 11 year old boy who survived and his leg healed without needing an amputation [7]. "*But when it had been shown by the researches of Pasteur that the septic property of the atmosphere depended, not on the oxygen or any gaseous constituent, but on minute organisms suspended in it, which owed their energy to their vitality, it occurred to me that decomposition in the injured part might be avoided without excluding the air, by applying as a dressing some material capable of destroying the life of the floating particle*" [7]. Lister treated 11 patients with compound fractures during this period and nine recovered [8]. He began to become bolder and started to treat all of his postoperative wounds with antiseptics. He treated bladder stones with suprapubic cystotomy and drained a perinephric psoas abscess all using his aseptic methods. In August 1867 at the Dublin meeting of the British Medical Association he announced that during the last 9 months "*his wards- previously amongst the unhealthiest in the whole surgical division of the Glasgow Royal Infirmary- had been entirely free from hospital sepsis.*" He published a series of five articles in *The Lancet* from March through July of 1867 and was asked to return to Edinburgh in 1869 to take his friend and mentor's place [9]. Anecdotally, it is interesting that Lister, while still a student in London, was present in December 1846 when Robert Liston, a renowned surgeon for his speed, performed the first major surgery in Britain under ether anesthesia [5].

At about 8:15 am on October 16, 1846 William Thomas Green Morton, an American dentist arrived 15 min late for destiny. He had been hurriedly trying to collect his new glass inhaler from a local glassmaker. The surgeon, Dr. John Collins Warren, was waiting with thinly veiled pessimism for Morton to demonstrate inhalational anesthesia on his patient, Mr. Edward Gilbert, who had a neck tumor at the Bullfinch Building of the Massachusetts General Hospital. It was recorded that Warren had exclaimed, "*Dr. Morton has failed to appear and I presume he is otherwise engaged*" [10]. Morton arrived just in time and Dr. Warren noted, "*Well sir, your patient is ready*." With this Morton applied his mouthpiece to Mr. Gilbert and in about 3 min, first replied to Warren, "*Your patient is ready, Doctor*." After completing the operation, Warren said to the watching crowd, "*Gentlemen, this is no humbug*!" [10] When Morton died at the age of 48 in 1868, Dr. Jacob Bigelow wrote his epitaph, "*William T.G. Morton, inventor and revealer of anesthetic inhalation, by whom pain in surgery was averted and annulled, before whom in all time surgery was agony, since whom science has control of pain*" [10]. Anesthesia was heralded as the "*greatest gift ever made to suffering humanity*" by the tabloids but it engendered a raging controversy regarding precedence. "*The extraordinary controversy which has raged, and which re-rages every few years, on the question as to whom the world is indebted for the introduction of anesthesia, illustrates the absence of true historical perspective and a failure to realize just what priority means in the case of great discovery*" [11]. After Liston's first case, the People's Journal of London declared, "*Oh, what delight for every feeling heart to find the new year ushered in with the announcement of this noble discovery of the power to still these sense of pain, and veil the eye and memory from all the horrors of an operation…WE HAVE CONQUERED PAIN*" [10]. Other agents quickly followed: chloroform (1847, Sir Ivan Magill intubated the trachea), cyclopropane gas and sodium pentothal (Ralph Milton Waters of Madison, WI) was the next major advance, no longer did the patient need to even be aware of the "gas mask" covering his or her face [12]. The alleviation of the pain of surgery, allowed Lister to develop a safer approach to large bladder stones and removal of foreign bodies [13]. W.E. Henley penned in 1870 after having an amputation performed by Lister:

> Behold me waiting- waiting for the knife.
> A little while, and at a leap I storm
> The thick, sweet mystery of chloroform,
> The drunken dark, little death-in-life. [14]

Or perhaps more skeptically, George Bernard Shaw speculated, "*Chloroform has done a lot of mischief. It's enabled every fool to be a surgeon*" [15]. In one stroke, the necessity of speed over method had been eliminated.

Let us look to the hallowed halls of Johns Hopkins Hospital and more precisely as to why H. L. Menken would rate William Stewart Halsted so highly in this star studded cast. Lister's methods took more of a circuitous pathway to success than did anesthesia. Though there were many ardent supporters, there were also detractors, but a small group of young New York surgeons carefully began to adopt the aseptic technique in the United States and one of them was William Stewart Halsted (1852–1922). Halsted began to experiment on the novel local anesthetic agent, cocaine (first used by Freud) and he and his young colleagues all became addicted to this narcotic. Halsted's life changed profoundly as he went from an outgoing, charismatic young surgeon and outstanding instructor to a gruff, taciturn, isolated perfectionist [16]. Throughout this period he continued his brilliant researches in surgery and surgical techniques and he was supported by Osler and Welch [17]. His protégés literally changed the face of surgery; Harvey Cushing became the father of neurosurgery and Hugh Young the father of American Urology. Surgical training in the United States developed the scientific flavor of the German model, Billroth and

Kocher were two great friends of Halsted's other than his faithful dachshunds, Nip and Tuck [16]. Halsted literally transformed our image of the modern surgical arena. He introduced surgical gowns that were boiled and sterilized. Special caps were worn to keep bacteria from falling on the surgical field. He next introduced the sterile, but reusable surgical rubber gloves that historically are linked to his scrub nurse, Miss Hampton who later became Mrs. Halsted [17]. The picture of modern surgery was almost complete with only the masks missing [18]. Ureteral stone surgery was about to undergo a modern surgical epiphany.

Uroradiography

William Conrad Röntgen (1845–1923) was born on March 27, 1845 in Lennep, a small town on the Lower Rhine. He trained in the Netherlands but attended the University of Utrecht to study physics. He married Anna Bertha Ludwig of Zürich in 1872; they never had children of their own, but adopted a daughter of his brother's named Josephine [19]. His first published work concerned the specific heat of gasses, and he was also interested in the thermal conductivity of crystals. In 1895 he was studying the phenomena accompanying the passage of an electric current through gases of low pressure. He was following leads by many others, including Thomas Edison and Heinrich Hertz. He utilized a tube modified from Sir William Crookes that was initially described by Ruhmkorff. On the evening of November 8, 1895 he discovered that the tubes emitted another type of ray that passed through coatings. In fact he immobilized his wife's hand over a photographic plate and subsequently after developing the photograph noted his wife's bones of the hand with the ring she was wearing as a shadow image. He proceeded to perform subsequent experiments prior to publishing and presenting his findings on December 28, 1895. His paper was rapidly translated into many languages and *Die Presse*, a Vienna newspaper heralded the breakthrough on its front page of the Sunday edition; "*A sensational discovery of Professor 'Routgen' of Wurzburg has stirred the imagination of leading scientists*" [20].

Röntgen did more than sit on his idea, however. He proceeded to make a series of photographic X-ray impressions and sent them with a copy of his paper to other physicists who he knew were interested in this work. On January 1, 1896 Röntgen wrote to several of his colleagues and enclosed in some cases, at least eight images or examples of the very first radiographs each marked with the stamp "*Physik Institut der Univerität Würzburg*." He included the first of his three papers on X-rays. Röntgen's own attitude on his own work was one of caution. Sir Arthur Schuster a professor of physics at the Manchester University was one of the first English persons to receive this envelope. He noted "*I opened a flat envelope containing photographs, which without accompanying explanation, were unintelligible. Among them was one showing the outlines of a hand, with its bones clearly marked inside. I looked for a letter which might give the name of the sender and explain the photographs. There was none, but inside an insignificant wrapper I found a thin pamphlet entitled "Uber eine neue Art von Strahlen." by W C Röntgen.*" Soon Shuster would complain that "*my laboratory was inundated by medical men bringing patients, who were suspected of having needles in various parts of their bodies and during one week I had to give the best part of three mornings locating a needle in the foot of a ballet dancer.*" The firestorm had started and several textbooks on X-rays were rapidly published [21].

John MacIntyre in Edinburgh published his historical paper of the first clinical use of the new X-rays in a patient with stone disease on July 11, 1896 [22]. MacIntyre began, "*During the past four months I have, at the request of several physicians and surgeons, tried to photograph some cases in which the presence of renal calculus was suggested by the symptoms present.*" He reported that he at first tried to X-ray and photograph prepared stone specimens ex vivo. This already had been done however, by April 21, 1896 Félix Guyon presented a radiological appearance of urinary and biliary stones ex vivo [23]. MacIntyre then went into the clinical details, he had been asked to X-ray a patient of Dr. James Adams of Glasgow who had already had a stone with surgery and was again symptomatic. He apparently noticed a recurrent stone on his X-ray photograph after 12 min of exposure time. The surgeon confirmed the location and size of the recurrent calculus and a new era had dawned.

Swain followed MacIntyre and published a case of a patient with a calcium oxalate stone made by X-ray that measured 1 1/8 × 7/8 × 5/8 in. [24]. He predicted the rise of radiologic diagnosis in the management of stone disease. He also evaluated stones ex vivo and included biliary calculi. He called the ability to visualize a stone "irradiability" and created a table to demonstrate X-rays abilities to image a stone:

Specific gravity	Permeability to X-ray	Density of shadow
Calcium oxalate	Biliary calculi	Calcium oxalate
Uric acid	Uric acid	Phosphates
Phosphates	Phosphates	Uric acid
Biliary calculi	Calcium oxalate	Biliary calculi

One of the first textbooks on X-rays was Henry Snowden Ward's 1896 work entitled *Practical Radiography* [25]. An American textbook followed a bit later in the year by an electrical engineer, Edwin Hammer and a New York City physician, Henry Morton (*X-Ray; or, Photography of the Invisible and its Value in Surgery*). In their work, Morton and Hammer speculated rather presciently about many of the future applications regarding the new ray [26]. Morton would continue in the field and published *The Archives of the Roentgen Ray* beginning in July of 1897. David Walsh published the first medical textbook in 1897, *The Röntgen Rays in Medical Work*. He covered a large possible scope for application. Francis Williams from Boston published his 1902 textbook called *The Roentgen Rays in Medicine and Surgery*. Here he describes the possibility of diagnosing stone disease. In 1908 Mihran Kassabian of Philadelphia published his *Radiography, X-ray Therapeutics and Radium Therapy* where he also mentions genito-urinary applications [23]. This brings us to E. Hurry Fenwick's 1908 textbook *The Value of Radiography in the*

Diagnosis and Treatment of Urinary Stone. A Study in Clinical and Operative Surgery [27]. "*Two groups of professional workers are mainly concerned in a careful study of shadows cast by the Röntgen rays in the urinary tract- the operator and the radiographer. Both work independently and yet both are interdependent. The former cannot justly cast the responsibility of shadow deduction upon the latter, though he is dependent upon him for skill in shadow detection. The radiographer cannot be content with merely producing shadows: he must aspire to the knowledge of their causation, and to obtain this he must examine critically and learn from the work of the operator. Each must give: each take*" [27]. There is no better opening paragraph to a new era of diagnosis than this one. Fenwick delineated the course of the ureters trying to limit the risks of phleboliths (calcified venous valves in the pelvis) which had caused false negative ureteral explorations. His book has 11 chapters and is richly illustrated by 80 x-ray plates. At this early phase of radiography, this textbook is amazing and clearly points out the potential for changing the way stone patients are diagnosed.

A. Béclère followed the pathway set earlier by Swain and calculated the atomic weights of the elements that make up stones and also correlated this with the X-ray ability to visualize the stones [28]. He noted that of the various salts, such as carbonates, urates, and oxalates that the absorption of X-ray increases with the atomic weight of the salt. In order of their increasing capacity of absorption he listed the stones as follows: urate of ammonia, sodium urate, magnesium urate, potassium urate, and calcium urate. These were the greatest atomic weight salts, but he realized that the number of atoms and the molecular structure might also play a role in X-ray absorption. He realized that the majority of calculi that cast no shadows on X-rays were largely of uric acid. Calcium oxalate, phosphate stones, and calcium carbonate all were readily imaged. Cystine stones he noted cast a faint shadow. He even looked at rare xanthine and cholesterol stones and proved that they were akin to uric acid and were not at all imaged. He noted "*The X-ray never lies*; *it simply penetrates bodies in inverse proportion to their atomic weights- it is not the X-ray that is at fault, it is our interpretation that is at fault*" [28].

The urology groups at Johns Hopkins and New York Hospital followed as well. O.S. Lowsley noted that the most common causes for X-ray to fail in the diagnosis of stones are the following: [29]

1. Faulty x-ray technique
2. Motion or breathing by the patient
3. Presence of gas in the intestines
4. Overlapping the calculus over bone shadows
5. Obesity of the patient
6. Failure to make a complete cystoscopic examination with retrograde pyelogram
7. Inexpert interpretation of the plates

Harvey W. Cushing (1869–1939) who is considered the father of neurosurgery and a gifted writer, won a Pulitzer Prize for his 1926 biography of his mentor and idol Sir William Osler [30]. Cushing was born in 1869, the tenth child from a family with strong lineage of physicians and scholars. He had just completed his internship at the Massachusetts General Hospital in 1895 when Röntgen discovered the X-ray. Cushing helped develop the early X-ray program in Boston. On February 15, 1886, a mere 6 weeks since Röntgen's report, Cushing wrote to his mother "*Every one is very excited over the new photographic discovery. Professor Roentgen may have discovered something with his cathode rays that may revolutionize medical diagnosis.*" He and the house staff at MGH purchased their own X-ray machine and when he left Johns Hopkins it was rumored that he took the tube with him [31]. He certainly brought his radiographic interests with him to Baltimore and he helped junior house staff develop the first X-ray equipment at Johns Hopkins. Let us relate the first X-ray examination performed at Johns Hopkins in Cushing's own words. "*It was in the fall of 1896 that I went to Johns Hopkins and made the first roentgenograms that were taken there, with the aid of a decrepit and perverse static machine as big as a hurdy-gurdy and operated in the same way, by turning a crank. My first paper submitted for publication contained an account of a case of a gunshot wound of the spine with plates showing a bullet which a Baltimorean had planted in the body of his wife's sixth cervical vertebrae*" [32]. He apparently became the technician during the early years, despite his grueling schedule as a resident of William S. Halsted's surgical service [33]. Another Hopkins' man who also interacted closely with Cushing was Hugh Hampton Young. Young was given the role to develop genitourinary surgery by the Chief, William S. Halsted. Hugh Hampton Young's textbook of Urological Roentgenology appeared in 1928. Now radiology assumed its modern foundation in the diagnosis and management of stone disease [34].

At the Hôpital Necker in Paris the department of urology was strongly interested in stone disease and Félix Guyon helped promote the first X-rays of stones. By, 1897, the first four radiological laboratories had been created in Paris, and by Guyon's colleagues Théodore Tuffier and Janet introduced the ureteral catheters and X-rayed the patients. Joaquin Albarran (1860–1912) was a Cuban-born urologist trained in Barcelona but had come to work with Guyon. He developed a whole host of technologies to improve the radiologic diagnosis, including the first radiolucent catheters. Albarran was the first urologist to ever be nominated for a Nobel Prize in 1912 but he died just prior to the election [23]. Howard Kelly worked with finely waxed catheters prior to radiology that would become scratched or etched when encountering a stone [35]. The X-ray was a vast improvement over this non-specific methodology. By 1914, another urologist named Pasteau developed a marked semi-opaque centimeter scaled ureteral catheter. Contrast materials were thought of, the first utilized was air, oxygen, and carbon dioxide. In 1903 Wittek injected air into the bladder to better X-ray and identified a bladder stone. In 1905 Wulff and Albers-Schönberg in Hamburg injected air and bismuth into the bladder of a stone patient [36].

Then in 1906 the German urologists Voelcker, von Lichtenberg, and Czerny began to investigate opacification agents with a variety of compounds including bismuth, lithium, silver, and then thorium. By 1914, Albarran began to use their silver compound (Collargol®) to perform retrograde pyelograms [37]. Marcel Guerbet, a French chemist had suggested using non-toxic iodinated compounds to Albarran. A German compound Iodipin® from Merck Darmstadt was followed by Lipiodol®. Sodium iodine was used at the Mayo Clinic in 1923 by the pharmacist Rowntree to visualize the bladder on a syphilitic patient. Osborne and colleagues followed with a clinical trial with no great success, but Graham and Cole switched to iodinated phenolphthalein in 1924 [38]. Thorotrast® was a sodium-iodine solution for intravascular X-ray exams but it was found to be carcinogenic. Legueu and colleagues utilized it in the 1920s for retrograde urography. In Berlin between 1928 and 1929 the synthesis of a watersoluble iodinated contrast agent was undertaken by a young American urologist, Moses Swick who worked for Alexander von Lichtenberg. He was in Leopold Lichtwitz's clinic at the time and knew that Binz and Rath had synthesized a new benzoic acid iodinated material. He tried this new compound, Selectan Neutral® on rabbits and obtained intravenous pyelograms. Swick took the new material and tried it on humans [39]. Von Lichtenberg began the official study using Uroselectan® and the IVP became the mainstay for diagnosing ureterolithiasis [40].

The intravenous pyelogram (IVP) was the "gold standard" evaluation despite recent detractors favoring other methods. After the development of Uroselectan® Schering AG developed Uroselectan B® and then Diodone®. Bayer came out with Abrody® and the French developed a diiodinated molecule called Tenebryl®. By 1930, Coliez noted that improved imaging was possible with ureteral dilation and Zeigler developed an abdominal compression device to aid upper tract visualization [41]. Von Lichtenberg summarized all of these developments in 1931 [42]. IVP provided accurate size, shape, location, and functional data regarding the calculus and the kidney. In one recent evaluation, the IVP revealed unexpected findings in 42 % of patients and altered the management strategy in 60 % [43]. The modern era was ushered into existence by the introduction of CT scanning which has proved to be superior for ureteral calculus imaging to all other modalities.

From Ureterolithotomy to Stone Basketing

Surgery was now possible and stone disease was ready to undergo an epiphany. No longer was colic to be suffered, endured, when surgery offered a now painless, and less risky method of delivering those suffering with stones. Aseptic surgery rapidly reduced the postoperative mortality and morbidity from wound infections. Upper tract disease could be diagnosed with first with finely waxed catheters as demonstrated by Kelly, then increasingly with X-rays, and finally with intravenous pyelograms that could now accurately determine the size and location of the stone. But these massively successful methods did not all come at once. Many were the patients following the availability of both general anesthesia and aseptic surgical technique that would undergo surgery for an upper tract stone, with none being found. Aggressive surgeons were perhaps following the dictum of George Bernard Shaw.

In 1923, Herman Kretschmer summarized the knowledge of ureteral calculous disease into three distinct eras. First was the early time following X-ray introduction when patients were explored for presumed ureteral stones, and significant numbers of patients had none. Next, the era when ureteral catheters and retrograde pyelograms were done in suspected ureteral stone cases, but open exploration was again necessary with significant morbidity. He now describes the current trends of cystoscopic retrograde techniques [1]. Howard A. Kelly catheterized the ureters in most cases that he suspected a ureteral stone, even with good quality X-rays. "*It is our habit in catheterizing ureters in practically all cases to wax the catheter tip before its introduction. The wax on the end of the catheter serves the purpose of a tell-tale, revealing the presence of any stone encountered by it in its passage up the urinary tract.*" He discusses the nuances of ureteral catheterization for stones." *The catheter must be introduced into the ureter without touching the side of the speculum. Striking the metal makes a flat, smooth facet which cannot be mistaken for the gouge of the calculus.*" Once withdrawn, the waxed catheter is taken and examined in bright light with a magnifying lens from three to five diameters, looking for the tell tale scratches of a stone. Kirkendall described a method of adapting Kelly's technique of waxed catheter passage for catheterizing cystoscopes. He lined the outer sheath of the outer sheath of the cystoscope with a loose-fitting rubber tube which protects the catheter during passage [44].

Winsbury White in his 1,929 textbook *Stone in the Urinary Tract* devotes Chaps. 7, 8, and 9 to the diagnosis and treatment of calculus in the ureter [45]. He notes the percentage of stones presenting at different levels of the ureter as follows: lumbar 22 %, iliac 7 %, pelvic 51 %, and intra-mural 17 %. He too, did not depend solely upon the radiograph, he used Kelly's method of waxed catheter method. He begins "*There are three alternatives in dealing with a ureteric calculus: the stone may be left to pass by natural means, its passage may be aided by transcystoscopic measures, or it may be removed by operation*" [1]. In Young's magnum opus *Young's Practice of Urology, Based on a Study of 12,500 cases*, his table 48 in Volume II, displays the outcomes from their 116 cases of stone disease [46]. Ureterolithotomy was performed in only six patients ("3 well, 1 improved, 1 dead, 2 no reply). Kretschemer noted in 140 cases of ureteral stones, patients passed them spontaneously in 26 % of the time [1]. He also reported that stones 5 mm or less were the most likely to pass. Crowell presented a series of cystoscopic management of stones and reports on various methods of management. He used local anesthesia of 2–5 % procaine and injected the anesthetic up the ureter on impacted stones, occasionally injecting oil to get a catheter to slide by the stone. The catheters were tied in place and slowly exchanged for larger sizes daily until two No. 11's and one No. 6 are all in together [47]. Rapid dilation of the ureter was described by Bransford Lewis using metal dilators and bougies but noted a danger in pushing the stone back into the kidney. Bugbee recorded the success of cystoscopic treatment as 326 successes out of 347 cases and Crowell noted 88 successes in 98 cases [48]. Contraindications to cystoscopic manipulation of ureteral stones were described as stone sizes above 2 cm., impacted or encysted stones, acute infection and in cases where there is known disease in the bladder or prostate. Ravich reported on a personal series of 758 cases or ureteral stones in a private series. Only 48 patients passed their stones spontaneously, 456 passed the stone after simpler cystoscopic manipulations, 17 were advised to have surgery but refused, and 68 were required open surgery. His open surgical incidence was 11.2 % [49].

John Swift Joly also waxed eloquently on the management of ureteral stones in his Chap. 6 of *Stone and Calculous Disease of the Urinary Organs* [50]. Joly presented the incidence of bilaterality of ureteral stones to be 3 % but thought it could actually be higher in silent cases that present only as post mortem cases. He worried about small stones as well as large ones, "*A large ureteric calculus simply means that the stone has not given rise to obstruction, and that the function of the kidney above it has been more or less preserved. This is only relative, as rapid growth of the stone indicates the presence of infection, and the kidney sooner or later succumbs to the infection*" [51]. Joly also discussed methods that have been used historically to try to induce ureteral stone passage. He noted that Albarran recommended significant hydration. "*Diuretics have been suggested including citrate of potash, diuretin, theocin sodium acetate, weak tea, barley water, Vittel and Contrexéville water (mineral waters)*" [50]. Belladonna was recommended by some, but questioned by Macht, and he describes the use of papaverin injected subcutaneously recommended by Bachrach. Oral glycerin "*does not appear to have any definite action*" [51].

Bumpus and Scholl reported on 640 cases of ureterolithotomy from the Mayo Clinic and had an operative mortality rate of 0.62 % [52]. They discussed the imperative of knowing at the time of exploration the exact location of the concretion for planning the surgical incision site. They recommended an X-ray within 1 day of the surgery. They recommend an extra-peritoneal approach in all cases, and once the stone was palpated to secure it prior to incising the ureter to prevent it slipping retrograde back up the dilated ureter. Once removed they further recommended exploring the ureter with a bougie to insure that there are no further stones. They did not routinely suture the ureterotomy closed stating that it difficult to suture the ureter many times because of the inflammation. They recommended leaving a small drainage tube which is placed next to the ureter in the vicinity of the incision and generally removed after 48 h. Closing this discussion on ureterolithotomy with some comments by Frederic E.B. Foley, the inventor of the indwelling catheter seems appropriate [53]. He began with the following comments, "*In recent years, ingenious devices and methods have been perfected for the passage or removal of ureteral stones without resort to operation.*" You can almost anticipate at this point that he is going to decry the newer, less invasive therapies for a careful open alternative, like the naysayers to Civiale. "*There is much evidence that this attitude has carried too far and that the just purpose of such management is becoming subordinate to mere zeal for its use.*" We can follow his path throughout the article, but he believes that the open surgery itself can be modified; making what was a major open operation, far less incapacitating. "*Lumbar ureterotomy, as described in textbooks and as usually seen, is also a definitely major operation; it can and should be a relatively minor one. A method and technic for lumbar have been perfected and are described here that so minimize the operation that in this form it scarcely belongs to major surgery*" [53].

Despite the success of ureterolithotomy, urologists continued to tinker with stone basketing and the development of various baskets for extraction. W.A. Council of the Brady Urological Institute in 1926 developed a multiple-wire cage for the extraction of calculi. H.L [54]. Cecil in 1926 developed the first stone crusher [55]. It should be noted that in this era of blind-stone basketing we have little mention of the complications following stone manipulation, though it would be expected that many disasters did occur, including ureteral avulsion as well as sepsis given that this was prior to the era of antimicrobial therapy.

A number of modifications were made to the earlier extraction instruments. In 1929, Bransford Lewis improved upon his 1904 forceps by combining elongated jaws and modified scissors in his new extractor [56]. Moore in 1937 would publish his suggestion that ureteral dilation should precede efforts at extraction though few contemporary urologists would adhere to Moore's principles at the time [57].

The loop catheter was the next significant advance in ureteral stone removal. Ellik would be credited with encouraging its use in the United States. Ellik's nylon loop used for extracting ureteral calculi consisted of a thin ureteral catheter with a nylon thread attached to the end of the catheter [58]. Once the catheter was passed into the renal pelvis, the nylon string was pulled creating a loop which was used to snare the stone as the catheter was removed.

In 1958, the best wire instruments came out of Italy, when Dormia fashioned a flexible extractor with a wire cage of significant tensile strength but flexible enough to cause little ureteral trauma [59]. The instrument was designed for interchangeable filiforms, which were first advocated by Earl Nation in 1953 [60]. The combination of a long filiform and an atraumatic wire cage that was deployed through the flexible hollow stem made it the ideal extractor during this era. The methodology for ureteral extraction prior to the development of the ureteroscope and Mulvaney's ultrasonic fragmentation of calculi and the eventual development of lasers was dilation of the ureter followed by various snaring techniques [61]. This methodology is still used today as ureteral dilation is occasionally required prior to ureteroscopy and treatment of the stone (via laser lithotripsy or stone extraction). The Dormia instrument would form the foundation for the nitinol tipped stone baskets of today.

Development of Ureteroscopy

Bozzini developed his "lichtleiter" in 1806 for viewing orifices in the human body [62]. Desormeaux would develop open tube endoscopy to examine the bladder in 1867 [63]. Nitze and Leiter in 1879 would pioneer the first modern cystoscope [64]. Advances in optics led to better cystoscopes which when minitiarized would serve as the first ureteroscopes. Advances in illumination would play a significant role in improving the cystoscope as it evolved from indirect illumination to heated platinum wires followed by the incandescent lightbulb [63, 65].

The first ureteroscopic procedure was performed by Hugh Hampton Young in 1912 and reported in 1929. The procedure was performed during cystoscopy in a 2 month old child with dilated ureters due to posterior urethral valves. Advances in fiberoptics led to the development of flexible ureteroscopes. Victor Marshall would perform the first antegrade nephroscopy and ureteroscopy using a fiberscope during an open exploration to visualize the pelvis and distal ureter in 1960 and would be followed by Takagi and Bush in using early flexible ureterosocpy in the early 1970s [66].

Despite flexible ureteroscopy predating the reports of routine rigid ureteroscopy, the early flexible scopes were not widely accepted because of their limited working capabilities (no method of deflecting the tip and no working channel for irrigation).

In 1977, rigid ureteroscopy was reported independently by Goodman and Lyon using an 11 Fr pediatric cystoscope [67, 68]. Due to the larger caliber scopes at the time, ureteral dilation often preceded rigid ureteroscopy in order to accommodate the scope diameter. Smaller caliber rigid ureteroscopes were made possible with the development of the Hopkins rod lens system in 1960 [69]. Prior to this, endoscopic instruments consisted of a hollow tube with a distal objective lens, an ocular lens and a series of relay lenses. Hopkins' rod lens system replaced the air spaces with glass rods which led to a more durable design and more efficient light and image transmission.

Richard Wolf Medical Instruments designed the first endoscope specifically for ureteroscopy (13 Fr, working length of 23 cm) and its use was reported by Lyon et al. in 1979 in inspecting the distal ureter [70]. Perez-Castro and Martinez-Pinero in 1980, working with Karl Storz Endoscopy, reported the development of a longer ureteroscope that could reach the renal pelvis [71]. Originally, rigid ureteroscopes did not have a working channel for irrigation and thus they relied on forced dieresis to keep a clear visual field. The 1980s would lead to the development of rigid ureteroscopes with working capabilities. Small baskets were used through the working channels of these rigid ureteroscopes for stone extraction, however as larger intraureteral stones were encountered the need for intracorporeal lithotripsy became apparent. By integrating fiberoptic imaging bundles and smaller working channels, manufacturers were able to further miniaturize the ureteroscopes. The half-moon image distortion, which resulted from the slight angulation/bending of the ureteroscope shaft was not encountered with the flexible fiberoptic imaging bundles [72].

The development of fiberoptic image transmission is based on the principle of internal reflection which was first shown by Daniel Colladon at the University of Geneva in 1841 [73]. The internal reflection allows for the bending of light within flexible glass. In 1957, Basil Hirschowitz working with a physicist, Lawrence Curtiss, developed the cladding process to improve fiberoptic design [74]. In this process, the individual fibers within the fiberoptic bundle are coated with a second layer of glass. The second layer creates an interface between the two glasses producing more efficient internal reflection. There was renewed interest in the development of improved flexible ureteroscopes when the limitations of rigid ureteroscopy became apparent. With the addition of active deflection, adequate working channels and smaller diameter working instruments flexible ureteroscopy became widely accepted for the treatment of ureteral stones that could not be easily reached via ureteroscopy. Improvements in imaging culminated with the development of the charged couple device (CCD) by George Smith and Willard Boyle in 1969 for electronic video recording [63].

Extracorporeal Shock Wave Lithotripsy

The German aerospace firm Dornier played a pivotal role in the application of shock waves to stone fragmentation. Dornier engineers became interested in the pattern of metal fatigue that they found on their aircraft and hypothesized that they were due shock waves produced by supersonic aircraft as the waves were focused inadvertently by parts of the plane's fuselage onto other parts of the aircraft. Dornier would show that shock waves could be produced using an underwater spark discharge and from that developed the application of shock waves to fragment human kidney stones [75].

The mid 1970s would lead to the research of Ferdinand Eisenberger and Christian Chaussy who were able to show that focused shockwaves were sufficient for stone fragmentation initially in dogs. At the time radiographic imaging was used and preferred over ultrasound to help target the stones. The successful animal research would lead to the first patient treated with SWL with the HM-1 (human machine-1) lithotriptor on February 20, 1980 [75–77].

The HM-1 would be followed by the HM-2 lithotriptor which was a simpler machine to operate as the electrode could be changed without removing the patient from the water bath. With the success of the HM-2, Dornier would introduce the first commercially produced lithotriptor, the HM-3 in 1984. The success of the Dornier's HM-3 lithotriptor would stimulate other methods for the generation of shockwaves for kidney stone lithotripsy. Besides electrohydraulic-based lithotripsy, shockwaves would also be generated using electromagnetic membranes, piezoelectric crystals and focused lasers [75]. An ellipsoidal reflector was used to focus electrohydraulic generated shock waves from F1 (focus of an ellipse where the spark gap generated the shock wave) to F2 (the location of the targeted stone). A water bath was used in the HM-1 and HM-2 lithotriptors to provide a delivery mechanism for the shock waves from their generation at the spark gap to their target. However, once it was discovered that sufficient shock waves could be transmitted through membranes with similar acoustic density, the water bath was eliminated from future lithotripter designs. The efficacy of most lithotriptors using a dry shock wave source appeared to be less that the Dornier HM-3, likely due to the energy loss as the shock waves passed through multiple interfaces (the membrane of the water bag/cushion). The improvements in fluoroscopy would be pivotal in helping target the stone and over time ultrasound imaging would also be incorporated into many lithotripsy systems.

Intracorporeal Lithotripsy

With the development of the ureteroscope and techniques for basketing, the development of methods to fragment ureteral calculi was the next important step. In 1913 Wappler would make the observation that "when a spark is brought into contact with both the hard and soft species of bladder calculi, it causes them to disintegrate." [78] However it wouldn't be until 1950 when Yutkin would obtain a patent for the application of electrohydraulic shock waves [79]. Electrohydraulic lithotripsy (EHL), initially used to treat bladder stones, was essentially an underwater spark plug and was used to produce a shock wave from the spark as well as a cavitation bubble. Contact of the probe with the bladder wall could lead to bladder perforation. With a decrease in the size of the probe and shortening of the pulse widths, the EHL probe could be used in the ureter and in 1978, Raney used the probe to fragment ureteral calculi [80]. He passed a 9 Fr probe to fragment distal ureteral stones by passing the probe blindly up the ureter and was able to fragment 90 % of the stones attempted (however there was ureteral extravasation in about 40 % of the cases). As ureteroscopes and EHL probes became smaller (3 F and 1.6 F), urologists were able to expand the location of the stones treated in the urinary tract. However, even with modern techniques the EHL probe was still found to be associated with unanticipated ureteral injuries [81].

The first investigation of ultrasound for the destruction of urinary calculi was undertaken by Mulvaney in 1953 [82]. The ultrasound probe works by applying electrical energy to a piezoceramic plate which then vibrates at a high frequency. The metal probe attached to the plate transmits the vibrational energy to the end of the probe which can cause stones to resonate at high frequencies and break. The ultrasound probe causes minimal damage to compliant tissue as the tissue does not resonate with vibrational energy. Ultrasonic probes (2.5 Fr solid or a 4.5 Fr catheter hollow probe) were used with the rigid ureteroscope to fragment ureteral stones and was found to be an effective technique for the treatment of steinstrasse and large (>1 cm) stones.

The laser was developed in 1960 with ruby being the first medium used [83]. The term "laser" was an acronym for "light amplification by stimulated emission of radiation." The ruby laser emitted a wavelength of 690 nm and was able to fragment urinary calculi but produced significant heat that lead to tissue damage. In 1969, Anderholm showed that if a solid material was interposed between the laser beam and tissue, there would be absorption of the light by the solid and subsequent vaporization of some of the material would cause a shock wave [81]. This shock wave could be used to fragment stones. Neodymium, a rare-earth element, was used to dope a transmitting crystalline medium and produced a wavelength of 1,064 nm. YAG (yttrium-aluminum-garnet) was used as the crystalline medium leading to the development of the Nd:YAG laser, however the high energies needed to produce shockwaves lead to fragmentation and shattering of the fibers at the tip of the laser. The Holmium:YAG laser, a 2,100 nm infrared laser was developed with the advantage that it had a tissue penetration depth of 0.5 mm so that it would only cause tissue damage if it was 0.5 mm or closer to tissue surface. Its long pulse width led to cavitation effects that tended to drill into stones rather than producing solely a fragmentation effect [81].

The Antegrade Approach to the Ureter

Willard Goodwin, the eminent urologist and the first Chair of the Department of Urology at UCLA, was the first to place a percutaneous nephrostomy tube. In 1955, while trying to perform a renal arteriogram, Dr. Goodwin placed a needle into the collecting system of a hydronephrotic kidney. He injected radiopaque contrast, thus performing the first antegrade nephrostogram. He then left a tube to drain the kidney, thereby placing the first modern day nephrostomy tube. In his paper he illustrates the optimal site of puncture as five fingerbreadths to the midline of the "13th rib" if it were to exist [84, 85]. Dr. Goodwin's percutaneous approach would lead to the realization that a percutaneous tract could be used to access the kidney and this would open the door to the antegrade approach to treatment of ureteral stones.

By 1976, Fernström and Johansson were the first to describe a technique for extracting renal calculi through a percutaneous nephrostomy under radiological control [86]. Instruments used to extract renal calculi under radiologic control included the Dormia basket which was placed through a selecter device used to help aim and manipulate the basket once it was in the renal pelvis as well as the Randall's forceps used under fluoroscopy for stone extraction.

The Birth of Endourology

In 1978, Arthur Smith, would describe the first antegrade stent placement when he introduced a Gibbons stent through a percutaneous nephrostomy in a patient with a reimplanted ureter with a urine leak to allow the urinary leak to seal [87]. Dr. Smith would coin the term "endourology" to describe closed, controlled manipulation of the genitourinary tract. Dr Smith would write that once his residents read this title, they – along with some of the radiologists – immediately changed it to the "end of urology" [88]. However, as we know today, this was far from the truth. One of his early papers with Drs Zuniga, Clayman and Amplatz describes a series of 63 calculi extracted from 25 patients with a high success rate [89]. The main failures occurred in stones that could not be reached due to narrow infundibula or with stones embedded in swollen mucosa.

His collaboration with Kurt Amplatz, an interventional radiologist and medical inventor, would lead to numerous innovations which would further advance endoscopic manipulation of stones as well as further develop PCNL. Many wires and dilators still bear Dr. Amplatz's name today [88]. Much of the equipment we use today in endourology and for PCNL was developed in this era.

Take Home Points

- Lister's antisepsis applied by Halsted to surgery combined with Morton's anesthetic inhalation would revolutionize the field of surgery and were the basis for future success in ureteral stone surgery.
- From Roentgen's x-rays to the development of fluoroscopy, advances in radiology would play a pivotal role in the diagnosis and treatment of ureteral stones.
- We began accessing the ureter primarily through the bladder from wax-tipped catheters and blind stone basketing to directly visualized treatment via ureteroscopy. The development and the improvement of the cystoscope and its optics lead to the creation of and advancements in flexible and rigid ureteroscopy.

- The placement of the first percutaneous nephrostomy tube by Willard Goodwin would open the doors to the eventual antegrade approach for treating ureteral calculi.
- With the discovery of extracorporeal shock wave lithotripsy we no longer needed direct access to the ureter in order to treat ureteral stones.
- The innovations and technologic advancements in the treatment of ureteral stones and the birth of the field of endourology has allowed us to fulfill the Hippocratic obligation that "I will not cut for stone."

References

1. Kretschmer HA. The diagnosis and treatment of stone in the ureter. JAMA. 1923;80(20):1425–9.
2. Pepys S. The diary of Samuel Pepys. New York: Washington Square Press; 1964.
3. Moran ME. Urolithiasis: a comprehensive history. New York: Springer; 2013.
4. Rosenfeld L. Thomas Hodgkin, morbid anatomist & social activist. New York: Madison Books; 1993.
5. Fisher Richard B. Joseph Lister, 1827-1912. New York: Stein and Day; 1977.
6. Simpson JY. Hospitalism: its effects on the results of surgical operations. Edinburgh: Oliver and Boyd; 1869.
7. Lister J. On a new method of treating compound fracture, abscess, etc.: with observation on the conditions of suppuration. Lancet. 1867;89(2272):326–9.
8. Lister J. On the antiseptic principle in the practice of surgery. Br Med J. 1867;2(351):246–8.
9. Lister J. On the effects of the antiseptic system of treatment upon the salubrity of a surgical hospital. Lancet. 1870;95(2419):123–36.
10. Ash HL. Anesthesia's dental heritage. Anesth Prog. 1985;32(1):25–9.
11. Osler W. The first printed documents relating to modern surgical anesthesia. Proc R Soc Med Hist Med. 1918;11:65–9.
12. Snow J. On chloroform and other anesthetics: their action and administration. London: John Churchill; 1863.
13. Carpenter JG. Supra-pubic cystotomy for traumatism, with perineal drainage. Cincin Lancet Clin. 1901;46(85):169–74.
14. Henle WE. A book of verses. London: D. Nutt; 1888.
15. Shaw GB. The doctor's dilemma. London: Constable and Co; 1911.
16. Imber G. Genius on the edge: the bizarre double life of Dr. William Stewart Halsted. New York: Kaplan Publishing; 2010.
17. Bliss M. William Osler. A life in medicine. Oxford: Oxford Univ. Press; 1999.
18. MacCallum WG. Biographical memoir of William Stewart Halsted 1852-1922. In biographical memoirs. Nat Academies Press. 1994;63(17):151–70.
19. The nobel prize in physics 1901, Wilhelm Conrad Röntgen. 6/14/2012 http://www.nobelprize.org/nobel_prizes/physics/laureates/1901/rontgen-bio.html.
20. Kraft E, Finby N. Rontgen's discovery of X-ray and Lenard's priority claim. N Y State J Med. 1980;80(10):1623–5.
21. Mould RF. The early history of x-ray diagnosis with emphasis on the contributions of physics 1895-1915. Phys Med Biol. 1995;40:1741–87.
22. Macintyer J. Roentgen rays. Photography of renal calculus; description of an adjustable modification in the focus tube. Lancet. 1896;148(3804):118.

23. Moreau, Jean-Francois: one century of uroradiology in Europe: 1896–1996. Inter Soc Rad 06/14/2012 http://www.ishrad.org/media/raw/european_uroradiology_story_1_copie.pdf.
24. Swain J. The effect of röntgen rays on calculi. Bristol Med-Chir J. 1897;15:1–13.
25. Ward S. Practical radiography. London: Awbarn & Ward; 1896.
26. Morton WJ, Hammer EW. X-ray; or, photography of the invisible and its value in surgery. New York: American Technical Book Co; 1896.
27. Hurry FE. The value of radiography in the diagnosis and treatment of urinary stone. A study in clinical and operative surgery. London: J & A Churchill; 1908.
28. Béclère A. Bull de l'Acad de méd. Paris. 1930;104:227–30.
29. Lowsley OS, Kirwin TJ. Clinical urology. Baltimore: The Williams & Wilkins Co; 1940.
30. Cushing H. The life of Sir William Osler. Oxford: The Clarendon Press; 1926.
31. Gutierrez C. The birth and growth of neuroradiology in the USA. Neuroradiology. 1981;21: 227–37.
32. Gunderman RB, Seymour ZA, Harvey W. Cushing. AJR. 2009;194:296–8.
33. Bliss M. Harvey cushing: a life in surgery. New York: Oxford Univ Press; 2005.
34. Young HH, Waters CA. Urological roentgenology; a roentgen atlas of the genitorurinary tract with case histories & an outline of urology in its relations to roentgenology. New York: Paul B. Hoeber, Inc; 1928.
35. Kelly HA. On a method of post-mortem examination of thoracic and abdominal viscera through vagina, perineum, and rectum, and without incision of the abdominal parietes. Med News. 1883;26:733–4.
36. Webster E. X-rays in diagnostic radiology. Health Phys. 1995;69:610–35.
37. Pollack HM. Uroradiology. In: Gagliardi RA, McClennan BL, editors. A history of the radiological sciences. Diagnosis. Reston: Radiology Centennial, Inc.; 1996.
38. Osborne ED, Sutherland CG, Scholl AJ, Rowntree LG. Roentgenography of the urinary tract during the excretion of sodium iodine. JAMA. 1923;80:368–73.
39. Swick M. Darstellung der Niere und Harnwege im Röntgenbild durch intravenöse Einbringung eines neuen Kontraststoffes, des Uroselectans. Klin Wschr. 1919;8:2087–9.
40. von Licchtenberg A, Swick M. Klinische Pröfung des Uroselectans. Klin Wschr. 1919;8: 2089–91.
41. Gorelik U, Ulish Y, Yegil Y. The use of standard imaging techniques and their diagnostic value in the work up of renal colic in the setting of intractable flank pain. Urology. 1996;47: 637–42.
42. von Lichtenberg A. The principles of intravenous urography. J Urol. 1931;25:249–57.
43. Wrenn K. Emergency intravenous pyelography in the setting of possible renal colic: is it indicated? Ann Emerg Med. 1995;26:304–7.
44. Kirkendall BR. I. A new method of passing the wax tip. II. Modification of the technic of passing the wax tip. JAMA. 1915;65:1253–5.
45. White HP. Winsbury: stone in the urinary tract. Philadelphia: P. Blakiston's Son; 1929.
46. Young HH, Davis DM. Young's practice of urology. Based on a study of 12,500 cases. Philadelphia: W.B. Saunders; 1927.
47. Crowell AJ. Analysis of fifty cases of renal calculi, discussion. J Urol. 1924;12:425–7.
48. Bugbee HG. Primary carcinoma of the kidney with impacted ureteral calculus. J Urol. 1921;5:267–78.
49. Ravich A. A critical study of ureteral calculi. J Urol. 1933;29:171–84.
50. Joly J. Swift: stone and calculous disease of the urinary organs. St. Louis: C.V. Mosby; 1929.
51. Macht DL. On the pharmacology of the ureter: III. Action of the opium alkaloids. J Pharmacol Exp Ther. 1916;9:197–216.
52. Bumpus HC, Scholl AJ. Ureterolithotomy. Surg Clin North Am. 1925;5:813–27.
53. Foley FEB. Management of ureteral stone. Operation versus expectancy and manipulation. JAMA. 1935;104(15):1314–8.
54. Councill WA. A new ureteral stone extractor and dilator. JAMA. 1926;86:1907–8.
55. Cecil HL. Cystoscopic removal of ureteral calculi: presentation of a new instrument. J Urol. 1926;15:529–37.

56. Lewis B. A new ureteral stone forceps. J Urol. 1929;22:587–8.
57. Moore TD. Factors determining the management of ureteral stones. J Urol. 1937;3 7:1–11.
58. Ellik M. The looped catheter ureteral stone extractor: perplexities in its construction and use. J Urol. 1949;61:351–8.
59. Dormia E. Due nuovi apparecchi per la rimozione dei calcoli dall'uretere. Urologia. 1958;25:225–33.
60. Nation EF. Facilitation of passage and extraction of ureteral calculi. J Urol. 1953; 70:373–5.
61. Scardino PL. Endoscopic manipulation of ureteral stones. In: Landes RR, Bush RB, Zorgniotti AW, editors. Perspectives in urology, vol. 1. Nutley: American Urological Association; 1976. p. 83–98.
62. Engel RM. Philipp Bozzini—the father of endoscopy. J Endourol. 2003;17:859–62.
63. Moran ME. History of ureteroscopy. In: Monga M, editor. Ureteroscopy: indications & technique. New York: Springer Science &Business Media; 2013. p. 3–12.
64. Herr HW. Max Nitze, the cystoscope and urology. J Urol. 2006;176:1313–6.
65. Moran ME. The light bulb, cystoscopy and Thomas Alva Edison. J Endourol. 2010;24: 1395–7.
66. Marshall VF. Fiber optics in urology. J Urol. 1964;91:110–4.
67. Goodman TM. Ureteroscopy with pediatric cystoscope in adults. Urology. 1977;9:394.
68. Lyon ES, Kyker JS, Schoenberg HW. Transurethral ureteroscopy in women: a ready addition to the urological armamentarium. J Urol. 1978;119:35.
69. Hopkins HH, Kapany NS. A flexible fiberscope, using static scanning. Nature. 1954;173: 39–41.
70. Lyon ES, Bano JJ, Schoenberg HW. Transurethral ureteroscopy in men using juvenile cystoscopy equipment. J Urol. 1979;122.
71. Perez-Castro EE, Martinez-Piniero JA. Transurethral ureteroscopy-a current urological procedure. Arch Esp Urol. 1980;33:445.
72. Conlin MJ, Marberger M, Bagley DH. Ureteroscopy: development and instrumentation. Urol Clin North Am. 1997;24(1):25–42.
73. Colladon D. On the reflections of a ray of light inside a parabolic liquid stream. Comptes Rendus. 1842;15:800.
74. Hirschowitz BI. A personal history of the fiberscope. Gastroenterology. 1970;36:864–7.
75. Lingeman JE. Extracorporeal shock wave lithotripsy: development, instrumentation and current status. Urol Clin North Am. 1997;24(1):185–211.
76. Chaussy C. Extracorporeal shock wave lithotripsy: new aspects in the treatment of kidney stone disease. Munich: Karger; 1982.
77. Chaussy C, Brendel W, Schmidt E. Extracorporeal induced destruction of kidney stones by shock waves. Lancet. 1980;2:1265.
78. Shah J, Whitfield HN. Urolithiasis through the ages. BJU Int. 2002;89:801–10.
79. Denstedt JD, Clayman RV. Electrohydraulic lithotripsy of renal and ureteral calculi. J Urol. 1990;143:13–7.
80. Raney AM. Electrohydraulic ureterolithotripsy. Urology. 1978;12:284.
81. Grocela JA, Dretler SP. Intracorporeal lithotripsy: instrumentation and development. Urol Clin North Am. 1997;24(1):13–23.
82. Mulvaney W. Attempted disintegration of calculi by ultrasonic vibration. J Urol. 1953; 70:704.
83. Mulvaney WP, Beck CW. The laser beam in urology. J Urol. 1968;99:112.
84. Palapattu GS, Bloom DA, Smith RB, Boxer RJ, Goodwin WE. Educator, innovator and pioneer. J Urol. 2004;172:40–4.
85. Goodwin WE, Casey WC, Woolf W. Percutaneous trocar (needle) nephrostomy in hydronephrosis. J Am Med Assoc. 1955;157:891.
86. Fernstrom I, Johannsson B. Percutaneous pyelolithotomy. A new extraction technique. Scand J Urol Nephrol. 1976;10:257–9.

87. Smith AD, Lange PH, Miller RP, Reinke DB. Introduction of the Gibbons ureteral stent facilitated by antecedent percutaneous nephrostomy. J Urol. 1978;120:543–4.
88. Smith AD. A personal perspective on the origins of endourology and the endourological society. J Endourol. 2002;16:705–8.
89. Castaneda-Zuniga WR, Clayman R, Smith A, Rusnak B, Herrera M, Amplatz K. Nephrostolithotomy: percutaneous techniques for urinary calculus removal. J Urol. 2002; 167:849–53.

Chapter 2
Radiology Imaging for Ureteral Stones

Abdulkadir Tepeler and Stephen Y. Nakada

Introduction

Imaging methods play an essential role in the diagnosis, treatment and follow-up of patients with urolithiasis. Precise detection of stone burden and location and delineation of the collecting system, ureteral and surrounding organs' anatomy may affect the selection of the treatment modality. The selection of the proper imaging method should be made individually. While plain radiographic studies are not favored methods for radiolucent stones, more detailed studies may be required for patients with anatomical abnormalities. Contrast studies are not preferred for patients with renal failure or with an allergy to contrast material. Children and especially pregnant patients who are more sensitive to ionizing radiation also require special attention. In this chapter the imaging methods used for ureteral calculi are summarized.

Plain Abdominal Radiograph

The major advantage of plain radiography of the kidney, ureters and bladder (KUB) is assessing whether the stone is radio-opaque or not. While most calcium containing stones (calcium oxalate monohydrate, calcium oxalate dihydrate, and calcium phosphates) are easily visible, struvite, apatite and cystine stones are semi-opaque and faintly visible on KUB. The radiolucent stones (uric acid, ammonium urate, and xanthine) are not seen on KUB unless they are mixed composition. Therefore, in some

A. Tepeler • S.Y. Nakada (✉)
Department of Urology, University of Wisconsin School of Medicine and Public Health, Madison, WI, USA
e-mail: nakada@urology.wisc.edu

S.R. Patel, S.Y. Nakada (eds.), *Ureteral Stone Management: A Practical Approach*, DOI 10.1007/978-3-319-08792-4_2

clinics KUB is routinely used in the evaluation of patients with renal colic. While it is valuable in the follow-up of patients with opaque residual fragments or in the reassessment of the location of opaque ureteral calculi, it fails to detect non-opaque calculi. Because of its low sensitivity (45–58 %) and specificity (69–77 %) rates, KUB is not accepted as a proper imaging method for the initial diagnosis of urolithiasis [1, 2]. Another study presented that KUB could demonstrate stones in only 59 % of patients who had a diagnosis of urolithiasis with computed tomography (CT) [1]. Based on this proof, Kennish et al. argue that KUB should be omitted as a primary imaging method for ureteric colic if CT is available [2]. They recommend KUB for additional imaging in patients with urolithiasis diagnosed with CT. In another study Lamb et al. demonstrated that treatment was altered significantly in 17 % of patients with KUB in addition to CT due to the detection of stone radiolucency or change in stone size and position [3]. Besides the evaluation of stone radio-opacity, the baseline KUB helps to image the bony structures, phleboliths and calcified masses that can mimic a stone so that it can serve as a baseline image that can be compared with future images.

The CT "scout" film (screening digital radiograph) is obtained during axial CT scan simulating KUB. Studies evaluating both imaging methods show that the stone visibility rate on the CT scout (17–49 %) is significantly lower than the rate of KUB (40–63 %, $p<0.001$) [4, 5]. Reduced contrast between stone and soft tissue resulting from lower spatial resolution and the high kilovoltage settings of CT scout leads to a decrease in sensitivity and specificity of CT scout in the detection of ureteral calculi [5]. Although KUB is recommended only if the stone is not visualized on CT scout, Foel and colleagues presented that definitive assessment rates increase with KUB and CT [6, 7]. Therefore, they recommend baseline KUB for patients with ureteral stones diagnosed with CT.

Plain X-ray (KUB) is a proper imaging method for follow-up for opaque ureteral stones having the advantages of being lower cost and less radiation exposure (0.5–1 millisievert (mSv) dose of radiation exposure) when compared to computed tomography [7].

Ultrasonography

Ultrasonography (US) is a common imaging method used by urologists because it is cost-effective, radiation free, non-invasive and repeatable [7]. The sensitivity of US in detecting urolithiasis varies in the range of 19–96 % [8]. While the sensitivity and specificity are higher for stones located in the renal pelvis, renal calices, the ureteropelvic junction, and the ureterovesical junction, detection of ureteral calculi is more difficult and requires expertise. The deep location of the mid ureter and presence of intestinal gas may hinder the visualization of the ureter and calculi. However, the stone might be detected by re-examination with US due to the migration of the stone to the distal portion of the ureter which is more visible. Therefore, US can be used for follow-up in patients with ureteral calculi.

In a study comparing the diagnostic accuracy of CT, intravenous urography (IVU), and US for ureteral calculi, the sensitivity was found to be 94, 52, and 19 %, respectively [9]. US may also detect secondary signs (hydronephrosis, ureteral dilation, lack of ureteral jet flow) that may be related to obstruction or stricture. To increase the accuracy of US, a combination of KUB and Doppler US is described in the literature. It is shown that KUB or Doppler US, in addition to US, increases sensitivity (79–97 %) and specificity (91–100 %) in the detection of ureteral calculi [10]. For radiopaque stone formers, combining US and KUB is regarded as an optimal imaging modality [9].

The twinkling sign, a sonographic artifact behind the stone detected using Doppler US, increases the detection rate of ureteral calculi [11]. Similarly, native tissue harmonic imaging (NTHI), a new sonographic technique, provides higher image quality and precise measurement of stone size. It gives more details even in obese patients [12]. Mitterberger et al. presented that KUB with NTHI-US has a comparable specificity and sensitivity rate with CT in the detection of urolithiasis [12].

Lack of radiation exposure and contrast administration, widespread availability and low cost are the main advantages of US. However, the requirement of expertise and low sensitivity for mid ureter, especially in obese patients, are regarded as limitations. Because of this, US is used as the primary imaging method in children and pregnant patients [7, 8]. Additionally, it is recommended as the first step imaging modality for the follow-up of patients treated with SWL or URS or in symptomatic patients who passed the stone to assess the relief of the obstruction [8].

Intravenous Urography

Regarded as the traditional imaging method used for the diagnosis of acute flank pain, intravenous urography provides information about renal function, the grade of hydro-ureteronephrosis, stone location, anatomical abnormalities of the pelvicaliceal system and ureter, and tumors in the collecting system and ureter. On the other hand, non-visualization of radiolucent stones with X-ray and difficulty differentiating the filling defect sign from other etiologies (e.g. urothelial tumors) are regarded as its major limitations. The requirement of a contrast medium injection, proper bowel preparation and adequate hydration are other concerns about the method. The administration of contrast may lead to contrast nephrotoxicity, a 5–10 % risk of allergic reaction, and the most severe complication of an anaphylactic reaction, with the risk of 1/100,000 [8]. The IVU procedure may be more time consuming due to the requirement of delayed films in patients with delayed urinary extraction related to obstruction. Chen et al. presented that room time for IVU was almost three times higher than the time for CT scan [13].

With the introduction of CT for the assessment of flank pain, the utility of IVU is significantly decreased. The studies prospectively comparing CT and IVU in patients with flank pain presented that the sensitivity and specificity of IVU (51–87 %, 92–100 %, respectively) are significantly lower than those of CT

(94–100 %, 92–100 %, respectively) ($p = 0.015$) [7, 14]. With the widespread availability of CT in emergency rooms, it has replaced IVU for the radiological evaluation of patients with acute flank pain.

Contrast studies can be helpful in the assessment of obstruction and renal function after treatment of a ureteral stone. Although the ureteral stricture rate after URS (1–4 %) and SWL (0–2 %) is reported to be very low, contrast studies (IVU, diuretic renography or contrast CT) can be used in the assessment of patients who have symptoms or persistent hydronephrosis after definitive treatment [8].

Computed Tomography

The usage of unenhanced helical CT for the diagnosis of acute flank pain was initially reported by Smith et al. in 1995 [15]. In recent years with its widespread usage, computed tomography, is regarded as the gold standard imaging method for the initial diagnosis of acute ureteric colic because it has the highest sensitivity (94–100 %) and specificity (92–100 %) rates among imaging modalities [7, 8]. The ability to diagnose non-urologic conditions mimicking renal colic, such as appendicitis, diverticulitis, pancreatitis, cholelithiasis, and lumbar discitis, its short examination time, and its high sensitivity and specificity rates make it the most useful and common imaging method utilized in emergency rooms.

The determination of precise stone size is essential in decision making for the proper treatment of ureteral calculi. While ureteral stones <5 mm have the spontaneous passage rate of 77 %, only 39 % of the ureteral calculi >7 mm pass spontaneously [16]. While KUB may lead to overestimation of stone size by 20 %, measurement with CT is closer to the actual stone size. However, Kishore et al. could not show significant correlation between actual stone size and CT measurement for distal ureteral stones [17].

Computed tomography reveals other stone related parameters [number of calculi, stone location, stone volume, stone attenuation measured in Hounsfield units (HU), and skin-to-stone distance (SSD)] that affect the selection of the proper treatment regime, in order to achieve the best results. Hounsfield unit attenuation and SSD are important factors affecting the success of SWL. Pareek et al. presented that SSD measured on CT is a powerful predictor of the success of SWL for renal calculi [18]. In this study, SSD of >10 cm was found to be the most sensitive and specific point on the curve, illustrating the relationship of the success of SWL with SSD. Stone volume measured using a three-dimensional (3D) reconstruction of the preoperative CT is also a predictor of success for SWL in the treatment of upper urinary tract calculi.

Hounsfield unit attenuation is another factor that can predict the success of SWL. Clinical studies have shown the threshold of stone attenuation detected on non-contrast CT for the failure of SWL was found to be >1,000 HU [7, 8, 19]. Some researchers made attempts to distinguish the stone composition using the HU measurements. Calcium based stones have a correlation between stone size and density, and they also have significantly higher HU attenuation than uric acid stones [20, 21]. Dual-energy CT (DECT) is a technique where scans at two different energy levels are obtained inorder to thereby allow differentiation in the composition of urolithiasis. In a recently published study, Wisenbaugh et al. have recently conducted a prospective and blinded study to compare accuracy of conventional CT and DECT in the prediction of stone composition [22]. They found that although both techniques have a comparable accuracy rate for the detection of uric acid stones, DECT is highly sensitive (93 %) in the differentiation of non-uric acid stones.

Another popular parameter measured on CT that can be used to predict the stone composition is visceral fat area (VFA). Zhou et al. measured VFA from a 5 mm axial slice at the umbilical level using software and examined the association between stone type and increased VFA [23]. VFA may be regarded as the reflection of visceral obesity that increases the risk of metabolic syndrome and urolithiasis. They presented that hypertension and increased VFA (>187 cm^2) are independent risk factors for uric acid. In another study the authors evaluated the association between parameters (SSD, HU, VFA) detected on CT and SWL success for ureteral calculi [24]. In their retrospective study, VFA (95 cm^2), total abdominal fat area (263 cm^2), para/perirenal fat area (49 cm^2), and SSD were detected as important markers for the prediction of SWL success. Further prospective studies are warranted to explore these parameters.

High radiation exposure is a major limitation of CT despite its high accuracy. A single abdomino-pelvic non-contrast CT leads to a 20 mSv radiation exposure which is approximately one third of the exposed dose of an atomic bomb within 3 km of detonation [25]. This dose of radiation exposure has the risk of radiation induced malignancy in 1/1,000 patients [25]. In order to reduce radiation exposure, low-dose CT can be used for the diagnosis of urolithiasis while having comparable sensitivity (97 %) and specificity (95 %) rates to conventional dose CT [26]. Jellison et al. showed that ultra-low-dose CT protocol produced an overall 98 % sensitivity and 83 % specificity for the detection of distal ureteral calculi with a 95 % decrease in radiation exposure [27]. Low-dose CT also provides reliable information about stone size, SSD and stone density. Besides its advantage in decreasing radiation exposure, low-dose protocol CT has less sensitivity in patients with a BMI >30 kg/m^2 and for ureteral calculi <3 mm [7, 8]. Although US is the primary imaging modality for the pediatric population when diagnosing urolithiasis, low-dose CT is considered if US fails to make a diagnosis when ureteral calculi are suspected [8]. For non-opaque ureteral calculi diagnosed initially with CT, low-dose CT has emerged as a proper imaging modality for patients whose symptoms persist despite therapy or observation [8]. Low-dose CT is also recommended after definitive therapy (SWL, URS or MET) to assess the symptomatic patients who have persistent hydronephrosis detected with US [8].

Magnetic Resonance Imaging

Magnetic resonance imaging is a radiation free imaging modality providing a comprehensive image for the assessment of all soft tissues. Although decreased sensitivity for the detection of urinary calculi compared to CT is regarded as a major limitation, secondary signs of urolithiasis can be detected with MRI. Generally, signal generating substances, including protons, become visible on MRI. While calculi are visible in low signal intensity because of their composition, the surrounding urine is visible in high signal intensity on T2 weighted sequences. The sensitivity of MRI depends on the stone size and volume of urine surrounding the stone. Gadolinium enhanced excretory phase imaging helps to visualize the stone by forming a contrast void between the stone and urine.

The MRI provides detailed information including hydronephrosis, ureteral wall thickness, and edema. Fegan et al. presented that the combination of MRI and KUB can diagnose calculus obstruction with a similar accuracy rate to CT [28]. Half Fourier single-shot turbo spin-echo (HASTE) MR urography provides faster image acquisition than conventional MR and does not require contrast administration. HASTE MR Urography is presented as an X-ray free and effective imaging method for the assessment of pregnant patients with suspicious renal colic [29]. While US is the initially preferred imaging method for those who are pregnant, MRI is regarded as the alternative method [7]. On the other hand, use of low-dose CT is allowed for the evaluation of flank pain in the 2nd and 3rd trimesters of pregnancy when US is not diagnostic [30].

Low sensitivity and specificity, increased cost, time consuming image acquisition, and limited availability make the MRI a rarely used imaging method for the evaluation of patients with urolithiasis. Because of its major advantage of being radiation free it is primarily used for pregnant women.

Take Home Points

- Imaging modalities are indispensable components in the selection of proper treatment strategy and follow-up for patients with urolithiasis.
- Urologists must be aware of the advantages and limitations of the various imaging modalities (Ultrasound, KUB, Non-contrast CT-scan, MRI) used to diagnosis a ureteral calculus.
- A number of CT-scan parameters may be used to help select the optimal treatment option for a ureteral stone including skin-to-stone distance and Hounsfield unit attenuation.
- Urologists should understand the radiation dose imparted by various imaging modalities so that the appropriate imaging test may be selected for the diagnosis and follow-up of ureteral stones.

References

1. Levine JA, Neitlich J, Verga M, Dalrymple N, Smith RC. Ureteral calculi in patients with flank pain: correlation of plain radiography with unenhanced helical CT. Radiology. 1997; 204(1):27–31.
2. Kennish SJ, Bhatnagar P, Wah TM, Bush S, Irving HC. Is the KUB radiograph redundant for investigating acute ureteric colic in the non-contrast enhanced computed tomography era? Clin Radiol. 2008;63(10):1131–5.

3. Lamb AD, Wines MD, Mousa S, Tolley DA. Plain radiography still is required in the planning of treatment for urolithiasis. J Endourol. 2008;22(10):2201–5.
4. Johnston R1, Lin A, Du J, Mark S. Comparison of kidney-ureter-bladder abdominal radiography and computed tomography scout films for identifying renal calculi. BJU Int. 2009;104(5):670–3.
5. Assi Z, Platt JF, Francis IR, Cohan RH, Korobkin M. Sensitivity of CT scout radiography and abdominal radiography for revealing ureteral calculi on helical CT: implications for radiologic follow-up. AJR Am J Roentgenol. 2000;175(2):333–7.
6. Foell K, Ordon M, Ghiculete D, Lee JY, Honey RJ, Pace K. Does a baseline KUB help facilitate stone management in patients presenting to the emergency department with renal colic? J Endourol. 2013, epub Oct 9 2013.
7. Turk C, Knoll T, Petrik A, Sarica K, Skolarikos A, Straub M, Seitz C, European Association of Urology. Guidelines on urolithiasis. 2014. http://www.uroweb.org/gls/pdf/18_Urolithiasis.pdf.
8. Fulgham PF, Assimos DG, Pearle MS, Preminger GM. Clinical effectiveness protocols for imaging in the management of ureteral calculous disease: AUA technology assessment. J Urol. 2013;189(4):1203–13.
9. Yilmaz S, Sindel T, Arslan G, Ozkaynak C, Karaali K, Kabaalioğlu A, Lüleci E. Renal colic: comparison of spiral CT, US and IVU in the detection of ureteral calculi. Eur Radiol. 1998;8(2):212–7.
10. Ripollés T, Agramunt M, Errando J, Martínez MJ, Coronel B, Morales M. Suspected ureteral colic: plain film and sonography vs unenhanced helical CT. A prospective study in 66 patients. Eur Radiol. 2004;14(1):129–36.
11. Ripollés T, Martínez-Pérez MJ, Vizuete J, Miralles S, Delgado F, Pastor-Navarro T. Sonographic diagnosis of symptomatic ureteral calculi: usefulness of the twinkling artifact. Abdom Imaging. 2013;38(4):863–9.
12. Mitterberger M, Pinggera GM, Pallwein L, Gradl J, Feuchtner G, Plattner R, Neururer R, Bartsch G, Strasser H, Frauscher F. Plain abdominal radiography with transabdominal native tissue harmonic imaging ultrasonography vs unenhanced computed tomography in renal colic. BJU Int. 2007;100(4):887–90.
13. Chen MY, Zagoria RJ. Can noncontrast helical computed tomography replace intravenous urography for evaluation of patients with acute urinary tract colic? J Emerg Med. 1999;17(2):299–303.
14. Niall O, Russell J, MacGregor R, Duncan H, Mullins J. A comparison of noncontrast computerized tomography with excretory urography in the assessment of acute flank pain. J Urol. 1999;161(2):534–7.
15. Smith RC, Rosenfield AT, Choe KA, Essenmacher KR, Verga M, Glickman MG, Lange RC. Acute flank pain: comparison of non-contrast-enhanced CT and intravenous urography. Radiology. 1995;194(3):789–94.
16. Preminger GM, Tiselius HG, Assimos DG, Alken P, Buck C, Gallucci M, Knoll T, Lingeman JE, Nakada SY, Pearle MS, Sarica K, Türk C, Wolf Jr JS, EAU/AUA Nephrolithiasis Guideline Panel. 2007 guideline for the management of ureteral calculi. J Urol. 2007;178(6):2418–34.
17. Kishore TA, Pedro RN, Hinck B, Monga M. Estimation of size of distal ureteral stones: noncontrast CT scan versus actual size. Urology. 2008;72(4):761–4.
18. Pareek G, Hedican SP, Lee Jr FT, Nakada SY. Shock wave lithotripsy success determined by skin-to-stone distance on computed tomography. Urology. 2005;66(5):941–4.
19. El-Nahas AR, El-Assmy AM, Mansour O, et al. A prospective multivariate analysis of factors predicting stone disintegration by extracorporeal shock wave lithotripsy: the value of high-resolution noncontrast computed tomography. Eur Urol. 2007;51(6):1688–94.
20. Nakada SY, Hoff DG, Attai S, Heisey D, Blankenbaker D, Pozniak M. Determination of stone composition by noncontrast spiral computed tomography in the clinical setting. Urology. 2000;55(6):816–9.
21. Spettel S, Shah P, Sekhar K, Herr A, White MD. Using Hounsfield unit measurement and urine parameters to predict uric acid stones. Urology. 2013;82(1):22–6.
22. Wisenbaugh ES, Paden RG, Silva AC, Humphreys MR. Dual-energy vs conventional computed tomography in determining stone composition. Urology. 2014;83(6):1243–7.

23. Zhou T, Watts K, Agalliu I, DiVito J, Hoenig DM. Effects of visceral fat area and other metabolic parameters on stone composition in patients undergoing percutaneous nephrolithotomy. J Urol. 2013;190(4):1416–20.
24. Juan HC, Lin HY, Chou YH, Yang YH, Shih PM, Chuang SM, Shen JT, Juan YS. Abdominal fat distribution on computed tomography predicts ureteric calculus fragmentation by shock wave lithotripsy. Eur Radiol. 2012;22(8):1624–30.
25. Pierce DA, Preston DL. Radiation-related cancer risks at low doses among atomic bomb survivors. Radiat Res. 2000;154(2):178–86.
26. Niemann T, Kollmann T, Bongartz G. Diagnostic performance of low-dose CT for the detection of urolithiasis: a meta-analysis. AJR Am J Roentgenol. 2008;191(2):396–401.
27. Jellison FC, Smith JC, Heldt JP, Spengler NM, Nicolay LI, Ruckle HC, Koning JL, Millard 2nd WW, Jin DH, Baldwin DD. Effect of low dose radiation computerized tomography protocols on distal ureteral calculus detection. J Urol. 2009;182(6):2762–7.
28. Regan F, Kuszyk B, Bohlman ME, Jackman S. Acute ureteric calculus obstruction: unenhanced spiral CT versus HASTE MR urography and abdominal radiograph. Br J Radiol. 2005; 78(930):506–11.
29. Mullins JK, Semins MJ, Hyams ES, Bohlman ME, Matlaga BR. Half Fourier single-shot turbo spin-echo magnetic resonance urography for the evaluation of suspected renal colic in pregnancy. Urology. 2012;79(6):1252–5.
30. ACOG Committee on Obstetric Practice. ACOG Committee Opinion. Number 299, September 2004 (replaces No. 158, September 1995). Guidelines for diagnostic imaging during pregnancy. Obstet Gynecol. 2004;104:647.

Chapter 3
Radiation Exposure to the Patient and the Urologist

Michael E. Lipkin

Over the past three decades, there has been a significant increase in the amount of radiation people are exposed to from medical sources [1]. Much of this can be attributed to the increased utilization of computed tomography (CT) scans [2]. Over 60 million CT scans were performed in the United States in 2006, compared to just three million in 1980. It has been estimated that a total of 29,000 future cancers may be caused from CT scans performed in the United States in 2007 [3].

Patients with ureteral stones are at particular risk for radiation exposure from imaging studies, especially non contrast CT (NCCT). The utilization of NCCT to evaluate patients in the emergency department for flank pain increased from 4 % in 1996 to 45 % in 2007 [4]. A study evaluating imaging during an acute stone event found that patients undergo an average of 4 diagnostic imaging studies in the year following the event, including 1.7 CT scans [5]. In addition to radiation from diagnostic imaging, patients with ureteral stones often require surgical intervention, and radiation from fluoroscopy used in the operating room contributes to their overall exposure. Given the risks associated with patient radiation exposure, every effort should be made to reduce the amount of radiation patients with ureteral stones are exposed to from diagnostic imaging and in the operating room.

M.E. Lipkin, MD
Division of Urology, Duke University Medical Center, Durham, NC, USA
e-mail: michael.lipkin@duke.edu

S.R. Patel, S.Y. Nakada (eds.), *Ureteral Stone Management: A Practical Approach*, DOI 10.1007/978-3-319-08792-4_3

Table 3.1 Summary of reported patient doses from diagnostic imaging used in the evaluation of urolithiasis

Study	Dose range
Standard non-contrast CT	8–16 mSv [7]
CT urogram	9.73 mSv [10]
Low dose CT	1.4–3 mSv [7, 11–14]
Ultra-low dose CT	0.5–0.91 mSv [18, 19]
Plain abdominal radiograph	0.5–0.63 mSv [8, 20]
KUB with tomograms	3.93 mSv [8]
Intravenous urogram	0.7–3.93 mSv [8, 21]
Digital tomosynthesis	0.87 mSv [20, 22]
Renal scan	1.8–3.3 mSv [21]
Ultrasound	0 mSv
Magnetic resonance imaging	0 mSv

Radiation from Diagnostic Imaging

Computed Tomography

Non-contrast computed tomography of the abdomen and pelvis is considered the first line imaging study for evaluation of acute renal colic. The sensitivity and specificity of NCCT for the diagnosis of ureteral stones in a patient with acute flank pain has been reported to be between 95 %–98% and 96 %–98 %, respectively [6]. NCCT can expose patients to a significant amount of radiation. The amount of radiation a patient is exposed to from a NCCT of the abdomen and pelvis varies with the machine used and the protocol used. Standard NCCT performed for the evaluation of stones have effective doses ranging from 8 to 16 mSv [7] (Table 3.1). For comparison, a single plain radiograph of the abdomen and pelvis (KUB) has been estimated to expose patients to 0.63 mSv [8].

In addition to NCCT, CT with intravenous contrast is occasionally indicated in patients with ureteral stones. A delayed or urographic phase (CT Urogram) allows for evaluation of obstruction and helps better delineate collecting system anatomy. The recently published American Urological Association (AUA) recommendations for imaging ureteral calculi recommends CT Urogram in patients who have undergone ureteroscopic stone extraction who have evidence of hydronephrosis on ultrasound (US) or NCCT [9]. The radiation dose of a three phase CT Urogram has been calculated to be 9.73 mSv [10].

Low Dose CT

More recently, newer CT scanners and newer scanning protocols have allowed for "low dose" NCCT. There is no strict definition for what comprises a "low dose" CT (LDCT), however in general it is accepted that a CT dose <3 mSv constitutes a "low dose" scan [7]. There have been a number of reports evaluating LDCT [11–14]. In a prospective comparative trial, the sensitivity and specificity for detecting ureteral calculi were compared between a standard NCCT (7.30 mSv in males and 10.00 mSv in females) with a LDCT (1.40 mSv in males and 1.97 in females) [11]. The two studies had comparable sensitivities and specificities, with the exception of stones <2 mm. In these cases, the sensitivity of LDCT decreased to 68–79 % compared to 95 % for standard NCCT. In another prospective trial, LDCT (1.6 mSv in males and 2.1 mSv in females) showed similar sensitivity and specificity for detecting ureteral or renal stones compared to standard NCCT (9.6 mSv in males and 12.6 in females) [12]. The authors did find that the LDCT had decreased sensitivity in patients with a body mass index (BMI) >30 kg/m^2. In patients with a BMI >30 kg/m^2, the sensitivity for detecting a ureteral calculus was only 50 % with a specificity of 89 %. A third comparative study evaluating the sensitivity and specificity between standard NCCT and LDCT also found equivalent sensitivities between the two imaging modalities for the detection of ureteral calculi [14]. A recent meta-analysis of studies evaluating LDCT for the detection of urolithiasis found pooled sensitivity of 97 % and a pooled specificity of 95 % [7].

Although LDCT has been shown to be highly effective at diagnosing ureteral calculi, it does have limitations. As mentioned above, the sensitivity of LDCT decreases in obese patients [12]. One way to overcome this decrease in image quality in obese patients is to use automatic tube current modulation (ATM) which adjusts the gantry rotation time to optimize the signal-to-noise ratio. When comparing radiation dose for LDCT using ATM in non-obese and obese patients, obese patients were found to have a threefold increase in radiation dose (3.04 mSv vs 10.22 mSv, $p<0.0001$) [15]. Given these limitations, the AUA recommendations for imaging ureteral calculi recommend standard dose NCCT in obese patients with suspected ureteral stones [16]. A recent study also evaluated the ability of LDCT to detect uric acid stones in the ureter [17]. This study performed in human cadavers demonstrated decreased sensitivity of LDCT for the detection of uric acid stones, especially for stones ≤3 mm.

Low dose CT is an improvement in regards to radiation exposure over standard NCCT, however it is still more radiation than a KUB. A recent study evaluated the effectiveness of an ultra-low-dose NCCT for the detection of ureteral calculi [18]. The effective dose for the ultra-low-dose NCCT was 0.91 mSv which compares favorably to what has been reported for KUB (0.63 mSv) [8]. When compared to LDCT, ultra-low-dose NCCT was found to have similar sensitivity for stones ≥4 mm [18]. Even lower CT doses have been evaluated. In a study evaluating NCCT with doses of 0.5 mSv in males and 0.7 mSv in females, the sensitivity and specificity was found to be 97 and 95 %, respectively [19].

Plain Abdominal Radiography

Plain abdominal radiographs (KUB) are still used in clinical practice for the evaluation of ureteral stones. For radio-opaques stones, they can be used to follow patients who are on a trial of passage. The dose of a KUB can vary based on the machine and settings used. The reported doses have generally been low, between 0.5 mSv and 0.63 mSv [8, 20]. The use of tomograms increase the amount of radiation patients are exposed to. For a series of KUB and tomograms, including one scout KUB image and three tomographic sweeps, the dose has been reported to be 3.93 mSv, more than a LDCT [8]. Intravenous urogram (IVU) is still used to evaluate for obstruction in the setting of ureteral stone and to delineate collecting system anatomy. The dose of radiation from an IVU is primarily dependent on the number of images taken and the technique. Reported doses for IVU have ranged from 0.7 to 3.93 mSv [8, 21].

Digital tomosynthesis (DT) is a novel technology which recreates a number of coronal images from a single tomographic sweep. The study involves a scout plain KUB and a single sweep of the emitter. Digital software then reconstructs a number of slice images at different depths. The advantage of this technology is on each slice, overlying structures are removed to provide clearer imaging. The radiation dose for DT has been measured in a phantom model to be 0.87 mSv which is slightly more than a KUB but significantly less than traditional KUB with tomograms [20, 22].

Nuclear Medicine Scans

Renal scans can be useful to evaluate for obstruction and determine differential function of patients with urolithiasis. The radiation exposure to the patient varies with the isotope used. The exposure from a renal scan with MAG3, DMSA and DTPA is 2.6 mSv, 3.3 mSv and 1.8 mSV, respectively [21].

Renal Ultrasound and Magnetic Resonance Imaging

Renal ultrasound is commonly used to evaluate patients with known or suspected ureteral stones. There is no radiation exposure from a renal ultrasound (US) which makes it the ideal first line study for pediatric and pregnant patients. Magnetic resonance imaging (MRI) is another imaging technique that does not expose patients to radiation.

Radiation Reduction from Diagnostic Imaging

Patients with ureteral stones are at risk for significant radiation exposure. The key to reducing this exposure is appropriate selection of imaging technique and use of radiation free imaging, such as MRI or US, as often as possible. The use of LDCT in lieu of standard NCCT also reduces the amount of radiation patients with urolithiasis are exposed to. The AUA clinical effectiveness review recommends

LDCT as first line imaging for patients with renal colic and suspicion for a renal stone with the exception of obese patients, in whom they recommend standard NCCT [22]. It also recommends a KUB at the time of LDCT and if the stone is radio-opaque, the recommendation is for US/KUB for follow up during observation. In general, the panel recommends US and KUB, depending on whether the stone is radio-opaque, for follow up after surgical treatment with shock wave lithotripsy (SWL) or ureteroscopy (URS). By following patients with US and KUB, the radiation dose is reduced nearly 80 % compared to if the patient had been followed with LDCT (0.6 mSv for US/KUB versus 3 mSV for LDCT).

Radiation Exposure in the Operating Room

Many urologic procedures in the operating room utilize fluoroscopy. This includes percutaneous nephrolithotomy (PNL), URS and SWL. The radiation from fluoroscopy contributes to patients overall exposure. It also leads to exposure for the urologist. Awareness of the amount of radiation patients are exposed to in the operating room (OR) and understanding techniques to reduce the amount of fluoroscopy will help minimize the overall exposure to both patients and urologists.

Radiation exposure from fluoroscopy can be reported in a number of different ways. Fluoroscopy time (FT) is the simplest measure of exposure, however it does not always correlate with the actual dose the patient received, particularly in obese patients [23]. Dose area product (DAP) is a value reported by the C-arm that can be converted to effective dose (ED) using conversion factors. Effective dose is a calculated dose that relates the amount of radiation absorbed to the risk of malignancy.

Percutaneous Nephrolithotomy

Patient Exposure

Percutaneous nephrolithotomy is often used to treat large proximal ureteral or uretero-pelvic junction stones. Fluoroscopy is commonly used to guide percutaneous access. In addition, fluoroscopy is used to help guide wires down the ureter, for tract dilation and at the end of the procedure to evaluate for residual stone and help with drain placement. A number of reports have evaluated radiation exposure and fluoroscopy time PNL [23–25]. In a retrospective review of 96 patients undergoing PNL, the mean ED was calculated to be 8.66 mSv [23]. Risk factors for higher radiation doses included increasing body mass index (BMI), increasing stone burden and increasing number of access tracts. Another review of 282 PNL procedures found a mean FT of 10.19 min [24]. In this study, increasing stone burden and access tracts was associated with increased FT.

Using a validated anthropomorphic male phantom model, one group measured organ specific dose rates and calculated ED rates for both right and left sided PNL in non-obese patients [25]. The ED rate was 0.014 mSv/s and 0.021 mSv/s for a right and left sided PNL, respectively. The authors retrospectively reviewed their series of PNL and determined the actual dose patients were exposed to by measuring the calculated ED rate by the fluoroscopy time for their procedures. They found a median ED of 7.63 mSv for right sided PNL and 8.11 mSv for left sided PNL. These doses are more than double that of a LDCT.

Surgeon Exposure

During PNL, the surgeon and OR staff are at risk for exposure to radiation from the C-arm. The primary risk for the surgeon is scatter radiation coming off the OR table or the patient. The majority of the absorbed dose that surgeons are exposed to is to the lower extremities, with the hands and head/neck getting exposed to lower amounts of radiation [26–28]. In one study calculating the ED the urologist is exposed to during PNL, the mean FT was 10.7 min and he mean ED for the urologist per case was 0.0127 mSv [28]. For comparison, the International Commission on Radiation Protection (ICRP) recommends that occupational exposure should not exceed 20 mSv per year during a 5-year period or 50 mSv in any single year [29]. In that same study, the absorbed dose the surgeon's eyes was exposed to was 40 μGy, compared to 167 μGy and 93 μGy to the lower leg and foot respectively [29].

Radiation Reduction

During any procedure using fluoroscopy, the principles of *As Low As Reasonably Achievable* (ALARA) should be followed (Table 3.2). These principles include ensuring the image intensifier is as close to the patient as possible and that the image is collimated over the area of interest as much as possible. Pulsed fluoroscopy

Table 3.2 Techniques to reduce radiation dose from fluoroscopy in the operating room (ALARA)

Technique
Collimate image to area of interest
Place image intensifier as close to patient as possible
Use pulsed fluoroscopy at lowest frames/sec that produces acceptable image
Use last image hold to save images for reference later in procedure
Use single shot fluoroscopy rather than continuous fluoroscopy as much as possible
Use low dose settings on C-arm where applicable
Use ultrasound when feasible (to aide in percutaneous access)
Use tactile cues in placing wires and place stents under vision
Have staff and surgeon stand as far from the emitter as possible
OR staff should use protective lead covering including aprons and eyewear

should be set at the lowest possible frames/sec that provides usable image quality to perform the procedure and last image hold should be used to save images for reference during the procedure.

In addition to adhering to the principles of ALARA, several other techniques have been shown to reduce radiation exposure. One group showed a mean FT reduction from 175 to 33 s using simple protocol during PNL [30]. The protocol involved marking the location of important landmarks on the drape, using a laser guided C-arm and having pre-operative imaging available and visible during the entire procedure. Fluoroscopy for access was timed during the end of expiration which is the longest period of the respiratory cycle. Another way to reduce radiation exposure to patients when fluoroscopy is used during PNL is to use air as a contrast agent instead of iodinated contrast [31]. The use of air instead of contrast was shown to reduce ED for almost 50 %, from 7.67 mSv to 4.45 mSv.

Another way to reduce radiation to both the patient and surgeon during PNL is to limit FT with the use of ultrasound to guide access. Two randomized controlled trials comparing PCNL with ultrasound combined with fluoroscopy versus fluoroscopy alone both found that the use of ultrasound reduces the FT by approximately 50 % [32, 33]. There have also been reports of using ultrasound without fluoroscopy during PNL, which completely eliminates any patient or surgeon radiation exposure [34].

In addition to the above recommendations, surgeon dose can specifically be reduced with appropriate shielding with lead aprons, lead lined glasses and lead lined gloves. Lead skirts can be applied to the side of OR beds reducing scatter to the surgeon. All personnel should stand as far from the radiation source as possible as the dose significantly decreases the further away the surgeon is from the emitter [27].

Ureteroscopy

Patient Exposure

Radiation from fluoroscopy during URS also contributes to the overall exposure of patients' with ureteral stones. The amount of radiation patients are exposed to during URS is less than that for PNL. In a study using a validated, anthropomorphic model of a non-obese male on a fixed fluoroscopy table, the ED rate for URS was calculated to be 0.024 mSv/s [35]. The median FT was 46.95 s and the median ED was 1.13 mSv, approximately the dose of two KUB. Obesity is a risk for increased radiation exposure during URS. Obese patients absorb a greater amount of radiation for the same FT as non-obese patients [36]. This is due to a feature of many modern C-arms called automatic exposure rate control which adjusts tube voltage and tube current to maintain image quality. Due to the increased amount of tissue to penetrate, morbidly obese patients have been shown to be exposed to more than three times the radiation as non-obese patients during ureteroscopy [36].

Surgeon Exposure

The reported risks of radiation exposure to the surgeon during URS are less than that during PNL [27]. Using a portable C-arm, the lower extremities are exposed to the greatest amount of radiation, with the head/eye getting exposed to relatively small doses. In a study evaluating surgeon exposure during ureteral procedures with a mean FT of 78 s, surgeons were eyes were exposed to a mean of 1.9 μGy, their lower legs to 11.6 μGy and their feet to 6.4 μGy. This would likely be different when a fixed fluoroscopy table is used. The x-ray emitter is typically housed above the patient in a fixed table unit. This would lead to scatter coming off the anterior surface of the patient, leading to greater exposure to the head/eyes.

Radiation Reduction

The principles of ALARA, as mentioned above, apply to the use of fluoroscopy during URS as well (Table 3.2). The best way to reduce radiation exposure to both the patient and surgeon during URS is to reduce FT. One study demonstrated a reduction of mean FT from 86.1 to 15.5 s by implementing a reduced radiation fluoroscopy protocol [37]. This protocol included the use of last image hold, use of tactile clues for guidewire placement, placing ureteral stents under visual guidance, and using a laser guided C-arm. The tracking of FT and providing feedback to surgeons has also been shown to be effective at reducing FT during URS [38]. Surgeons' FT was tracked for 9 months to establish a baseline. Thereafter, a quarterly report was given to all the participating urologists that included their mean FT and that of their colleagues. The mean FT decreased by 24 % once the quarterly reports were introduced from a mean of 2.74 to 2.08 min. The use of ultrasound to guide URS has also been reported, specifically for pregnant patients [39].

Shock Wave Lithotripsy

Patient Exposure

Shock wave lithotripsy (SWL) commonly uses fluoroscopy to target the stone during the treatment. Patient exposure during SWL is dependent on FT. One group evaluated the ED from SWL at their institution by determining the ED rate using a phantom model and then multiplying it by FT [40]. The authors found the mean ED to be higher for proximal ureteral stones compared to distal ureteral stones and higher for females compared to males. For proximal ureteral stones, males were exposed to a mean of 1.71 mSv versus 1.82 mSv, and for distal ureteral stones males were exposed to 0.76 mSv compared to 1.62 mSv for females. Another study demonstrated similar results with a mean ED of 1.62 mSv with a mean FT of 204 s [41].

Surgeon Exposure

The amount of radiation urologists are exposed to during SWL has not been specifically characterized. In general, since the urologist does not need to be at the patient's side while fluoroscopic images are taken, the dose should be lower than that for PNL or URS.

Radiation Reduction

The principles of ALARA apply to fluoroscopy during SWL (Table 3.2). Every effort should be made to limit FT. For surgeon exposure, the urologist should stand at least 12 ft at which point the radiation is equal to natural background radiation. The use of ultrasound to target the stone can also be used to reduce radiation exposure during SWL.

Take Home Points

- Patients with ureteral stones are at significant risk for increased radiation exposure from both diagnostic imaging and fluoroscopy used in the operating room
- Low dose CT protocols should be used in non-obese patients with flank pain for the diagnosis of suspected ureteral stones
- Radiation from fluoroscopy during surgical intervention can expose patients to as much or more radiation then diagnostic imaging studies
- Obesity increases radiation doses from both imaging studies such as NCCT and fluoroscopy in the operating room
- The principles of ALARA should be followed in the operating room to reduce radiation exposure from fluoroscopy to both the patient and staff

References

1. Mettler Jr FA, Thomadsen BR, Bhargavan M, Gilley DB, Gray JE, Lipoti JA, McCrohan J, Yoshizumi TT, Mahesh M. Medical radiation exposure in the U.S. in 2006: preliminary results. Health Phys. 2008;95(5):502–7.
2. Brenner DJ, Hall EJ. Computed tomography–an increasing source of radiation exposure. N Engl J Med. 2007;357(22):2277–84.
3. Berrington de González A, Mahesh M, Kim KP, Bhargavan M, Lewis R, Mettler F, Land C. Projected cancer risks from computed tomographic scans performed in the United States in 2007. Arch Intern Med. 2009;169(22):2071–7.
4. Westphalen AC, Hsia RY, Maselli JH, Wang R, Gonzales R. Radiological imaging of patients with suspected urinary tract stones: national trends, diagnoses, and predictors. Acad Emerg Med. 2011;18(7):699–707.

5. Ferrandino MN, Bagrodia A, Pierre SA, et al. Radiation exposure in the acute and short-term management of urolithiasis at 2 academic centers. J Urol. 2009;181(2):668–72; discussion 673.
6. Lipkin ME, Preminger GM. Imaging techniques for stone disease and methods for reducing radiation exposure. Urol Clin North Am. 2013;40(1):47–57.
7. Niemann T, Kollmann T, Bongartz G. Diagnostic performance of low-dose CT for the detection of urolithiasis: a meta-analysis. AJR Am J Roentgenol. 2008;191(2):396–401.
8. Astroza GM, Neisius A, Wang AJ, et al. Radiation exposure in the follow-up of patients with urolithiasis comparing digital tomosynthesis, non-contrast CT, standard KUB, and IVU. J Endourol. 2013;27(10):1187–91.
9. Fulgham PF, Assimos DG, Pearle MG, Preminger GM. Clinical effectiveness protocols for imaging in the management of ureteral calculous disease: AUA technology assessment. J Urol. 2013;189(4):1203–13.
10. Neisius A, Wang AJ, Wang C, et al. Radiation exposure in urology: a genitourinary catalogue for diagnostic imaging. J Urol. 2013;190(6):2117–23.
11. Kim BS, Hwang IK, Choi YK, et al. Low-dose and standard-dose unenhanced helical computed tomography for the assessment of acute renal colic: prospective comparative study. Acta Radiol. 2005;46(7):756–63.
12. Poletti PA, Platon A, Rutschmann OT, et al. Low-dose versus standard-dose CT protocol in patients with clinically suspected renal colic. AJR Am J Roentgenol. 2007;188(4):927–33.
13. Jellison FC, Smith JC, Heldt JP, et al. Effect of low dose radiation computerized tomography protocols on distal ureteral calculus detection. J Urol. 2009;182(6):2762–7.
14. Mulkens TH, Daineffe S, De Wijngaert R, et al. Urinary stone disease: comparison of standard-dose and low-dose with 4D MDCT tube current modulation. Am J Roentgenol. 2007; 188(2):553–62.
15. Wang AJ, Nguyen G, Toncheva G, et al. Radiation exposure from non-contrast CT, digital tomosynthesis, and standard KUB and tomograms. J Endourol. 2011;25(S1):A304–305.
16. Fulgham PF, Assimos DG, Pearle MS, Preminger GM. Clinical effectiveness protocol for imaging in the management of ureteral calculous disease: AUA technology assessment. J Urol. 2012;189(4):1203–13. [cited 2014 June 1]. https://www.auanet.org/common/pdf/education/clinical-guidance/Imaging-Assessment.pdf.
17. Huang GO, Engebretsen SR, Smith JC, Wallner CL, Culpepper DJ, Creech JD, Ng CC, Mai AT, Chung CS, Olgin G, Arnold 2nd DC, Baldwin DD. Detection of uric acid stones in the ureter using low- and conventional-dose computed tomography. Urology. 2014;4295(14):00180. epub April 17, 2014.
18. Pooler BD, Lubner MG, Kim DH, Ryckman EM, Sivalingam S, Tang J, Nakada SY, Chen GH, Pickhardt PJ. Prospective trial for the detection of urolithiasis at ultra-low-dose (sub-mSv) non-contrast CT: direct comparison against routine low-dose reference standard. J Urol. 2014;5347(14):03621–0. epub May 21, 2104.
19. Kluner C, Hein PA, Gralla O, et al. Does ultra-low-dose CT with a radiation dose equivalent to that of KUB suffice to detect renal and ureteral calculi? J Comput Assist Tomogr. 2006; 30(1):44–50.
20. Mermuys K, De Geeter F, Bacher K, et al. Digital tomosynthesis in the detection of urolithiasis: diagnostic performance and dosimetry compared with digital radiography with MDCT as the reference standard. AJR Am J Roentgenol. 2010;195(1):161–7.
21. Mettler Jr FA, Huda W, Yoshizumi TT, Mahesh M. Effective doses in radiology and diagnostic nuclear medicine: a catalog. Radiology. 2008;248(1):254–63.
22. Neisius A, Astroza GM, Kuntz NJ, et al. Specific organ doses utilizing a new technique for imaging nephrolithiasis: digital tomosynthesis. J Urol. 2013;189(4):e852, supplement.
23. Mancini JG, Raymundo EM, Lipkin M, et al. Factors affecting patient radiation exposure during percutaneous nephrolithotomy. J Urol. 2010;184(6):2373–7.
24. Tepeler A, Binbay M, Yuruk E, et al. Factors affecting the fluoroscopic screening time during percutaneous nephrolithotomy. J Endourol. 2009;23(11):1825–9.

25. Lipkin ME, Mancini JG, Toncheva G, et al. Organ-specific radiation dose rates and effective dose rates during percutaneous nephrolithotomy. J Endourol. 2012;26(5):439–43.
26. Geterud K, Larsson A, Mattsson S. Radiation dose to patients and personnel during fluoroscopy at percutaneous renal stone extraction. Acta Radiol. 1989;30(2):201–5.
27. Hellawell GO, Mutch SJ, Thevendran G, et al. Radiation exposure and the urologist: what are the risks? J Urol. 2005;174(3):948–52; discussion 952.
28. Safak M, Olgar T, Bor D, et al. Radiation doses of patients and urologists during percutaneous nephrolithotomy. J Radiol Prot. 2009;29(3):409–15.
29. International Commission on Radiological Protection. The 2007 Recommendations of the International Commission on Radiological Protection, ICRP Publication 103, vol. 37. Oxford: Ann ICRP; 2007. p. 1–332.
30. Blair B, Huang G, Arnold D, et al. Reduced fluoroscopy protocol for percutaneous nephrostolithotomy: feasibility, outcomes and effects on fluoroscopy time. J Urol. 2013;190(6): 2112–6.
31. Lipkin ME, Mancini JG, Zilberman DE, et al. Reduced radiation exposure with the use of an air retrograde pyelogram during fluoroscopic access for percutaneous nephrolithotomy. J Endourol. 2011;25(4):563–7.
32. Agarwal M, Agrawal MS, Jaiswal A, et al. Safety and efficacy of ultrasonography as an adjunct to fluoroscopy for renal access in percutaneous nephrolithotomy (PCNL). BJU Int. 2011;108(8):1346–9.
33. Basiri A, Ziaee AM, Kianian HR, et al. Ultrasonographic versus fluoroscopic access for percutaneous nephrolithotomy: a randomized clinical trial. J Endourol. 2008;22(2):281–4.
34. Alan C, KoÇoğlu H, Ateş F, et al. Ultrasound-guided X-ray free percutaneous nephrolithotomy for treatment of simple stones in the flank position. Urol Res. 2011;39(3):205–12.
35. Lipkin ME, Wang AJ, Toncheva G, et al. Determination of patient radiation dose during ureteroscopic treatment of urolithiasis using a validated model. J Urol. 2012;187(3):920–4.
36. Hsi RS, Zamora DA, Kanal KM, Harper JD. Severe obesity is associated with 3-fold higher radiation dose rate during ureteroscopy. Urology. 2013;82(4):780–5.
37. Greene DJ, Tenggadjaja CF, Bowman RJ, et al. Comparison of a reduced radiation fluoroscopy protocol to conventional fluoroscopy during uncomplicated ureteroscopy. Urology. 2011;78(2): 286–90.
38. Ngo TC, Macleod LC, Rosenstein DI, et al. Tracking intraoperative fluoroscopy utilization reduces radiation exposure during ureteroscopy. J Endourol. 2011;25(5):763–7.
39. Deters LA, Belanger G, Shah O, Pais VM. Ultrasound guided ureteroscopy in pregnancy. Clin Nephrol. 2013;79(2):118–23.
40. Perisinakis K, Damilakis J, Anezinis P, et al. Assessment of patient effective radiation dose and associated radiogenic risk from extracorporeal shock-wave lithotripsy. Health Phys. 2002;83(6):847–53.
41. Sandilos P, Tsalafoutas I, Koutsokalis G, et al. Radiation doses to patients from extracorporeal shock wave lithotripsy. Health Phys. 2006;90(6):583–7.

Chapter 4
Selecting the Appropriate Treatment Modality for Ureteral Calculi

Tim Tran and Gyan Pareek

Introduction

Urolithiasis is a common disorder that represents a significant burden to patients and the healthcare system. Three decades ago, the prevalence of urolithiasis in the United States was approximately 3.8 %. Since then, the prevalence has more than doubled, to a reported 8.8 % in a 2010 national survey [1].

Amongst patients treated for urolithiasis, nearly half will develop a second stone within 5–7 years [2]. Given this high prevalence and recurrence rate, it is not surprising that the national expenditure in relation to urolithiasis in the United States is over $2 billion dollars [3].

As one of the most common challenges encountered by the urologist, an in-depth understanding of the various treatment options for urolithiasis can facilitate safe and cost-effective care. The technological evolution in management options and its associated effect on treatment efficacy can make selecting the best option a challenge. This chapter aims to provide an up-to-date perspective on how to select an optimal treatment option for ureteral stones.

History of Ureteral Stone Treatment

Over the last quarter century, the treatment for ureteral stones has advanced greatly. Introduction of shockwave lithotripsy (SWL) in mid-1980s represented a revolutionary breakthrough. SWL offered urologists an effective and non-invasive

T. Tran, MD (✉) • G. Pareek, MD
Division of Urology, The Warren Alpert Medical School of Brown University, Providence, RI, USA
e-mail: ttran@lifespan.org

S.R. Patel, S.Y. Nakada (eds.), *Ureteral Stone Management: A Practical Approach*, DOI 10.1007/978-3-319-08792-4_4

treatment modality that featured less morbidity and a lower risk of complications than its contemporary counterparts.

At that time, ureteroscopy (URS) was typically limited to the treatment of distal ureteral stones. Poor optics, inefficient options for intracorporeal lithotripsy and larger instruments combined for a procedure that was wrought with technical difficulty as well as higher complication rates.

Subsequently, there have been significant advancements in URS. Miniaturization of equipment, ureteral access sheaths, improved fiberoptics, and deflectable tip flexible ureteroscopes highlight changes that have allowed for safer and more consistent access to the entirety of the upper urinary tract. The holmium laser has facilitated safer and more effective stone fragmentation. These advancements eased the learning curve for URS, leading to increased surgeon proficiency. Intraoperative complications, such as ureteral perforation and stricture, appear to have become less common with these advances.

The advancement of SWL over the last two decades has been less straightforward. Second-generation lithotripters have offered portability and decreased anesthetic requirements, however, stone-free rates have dropped considerably [4, 5]. A meta-analysis included in the 2007 Guideline for Management of Ureteral Calculi considered over 7,000 patients from 50 studies. Their findings noted that over a 10-year time period, the success rate of SWL for distal stones had decreased from 85 to 74 % [6].

The implementation of third-generation shockwave devices has yielded promising results. Over the last half-decade, stone-free rates with these lithotripters have been reported to approach or match the standard established by first generation devices, while maintaining the benefit of lesser anesthetic requirements. These results need to be validated in a more prospective manner. The constantly shifting milieu of ureteral stone treatment makes accurate characterization of the efficacy and safety of URS and SWL a challenging task. Further complicating this assessment is the paucity of high-level evidence to definitively compare these two treatment modalities.

Treatment Considerations for Medical Expulsive Therapy, Shockwave Lithotripsy and Ureteroscopy

Medical Expulsive Therapy

While the primary surgical options for ureteral stones are URS and SWL, medical expulsive therapy (MET) maintains an important role in management. Over the last decade, a series of studies have highlighted the importance of medical therapy in augmenting the successful passage of ureteral stones.

Preminger and colleagues have estimated that 68 % of stones less than 5 mm and 47 % of stones 5–10 mm are likely to pass spontaneously [6]. Based on these findings, a trial of MET is often a first line therapeutic option for ureteral stones less than 10 mm. Stone passage, however, can be extremely uncomfortable for the patient. As such, potential treatment options that can expedite the rate of stone passage and improve success rates may improve quality of life and help patients avoid surgery. More expeditious passage can also reduce the risk of urinary tract infection and obstruction-related deterioration of renal function.

The mechanism through which MET facilitates stone passage has been demonstrated in animal studies. The lodging of a stone within the ureter leads to uncoordinated ureteral spasm proximal to the stone. Alpha-blockers reportedly relax the ureteral smooth muscle to restore normal peristalsis and increase hydrostatic pressure proximal to the stone, facilitating distal progression of the stone [7].

The efficacy of MET on stone passage has been carefully examined over the last decade.

Agents that have been considered for MET include calcium-channel blockers, alpha-blockers and corticosteroids. In a meta-analysis by Hollingsworth et al. [8] both alpha-adrenergic antagonists and calcium-channel blockers were demonstrated to improve the likelihood of stone passage, decrease transit time and limit pain [8]. In contrast, corticosteroids had an inferior efficacy profile and are now rarely used due to their significant adverse effect profile.

More recently, a 2014 Cochrane Review decisively demonstrated the benefit of medical expulsive therapy [9]. Their analysis included 5,864 patients from 32 randomized controlled trials. Patients that received alpha-blockers had a 48 % greater likelihood of stone passage (RR 1.48, 95 % CI 1.33–1.64). Stone passage occurred, on average, 3 days faster (MD −2.91, 95 % CI −4.00 to −1.81). Patients receiving alpha-blockers also had fewer pain episodes and hospitalizations. No adverse effects were reported that led to cessation of therapy. Comparison between 1,647 patients that received alpha-blockers to 1,276 treated with calcium-channel blockers showed superior passage rates with alpha-blockers (RR 1.19, 95 % CI 1.05–1.35).

The use of MET remains on the rise, increasing by 68 % per year between 2002 and 2006 [10]. The 2007 Guideline for Management of Ureteral Calculi includes MET as a primary option for stones less than 10 mm. Thus, amongst patients for whom a trial of passage will be offered, the addition of MET is advisable. Periodic re-assessment of stone progression with serial imaging is indicated. A trial of passage is deemed a failure in the presence of persistent obstruction, failure of stone progression or intolerable renal colic.

Shockwave Lithotripsy

The current body of literature on SWL makes it clear that the most efficient approach requires careful patient selection as well as optimization of operative techniques. Because non-contrast computed tomography (NCCT) is often available prior to SWL, several CT-based metrics have been reported to predict treatment outcomes.

Stone Density

Stone density, as measured by Hounsfield Units (HU) has been described as a surrogate marker for stone hardness. Softer stones, such as calcium oxalate dihydrate and calcium phosphate are more readily fragmented by SWL in comparison to harder stones, such as cystine or calcium oxalate monohydrate [11, 12]. Measuring HU greater than 900 was a significant predictor of SWL failure in one cohort and stones with HU >1,000 required significantly more shocks to achieve fragmentation in another [13, 14]. Ouzaid et al. demonstrated a 96 % SFR for stones with HU <970, while those >970 had SFR of only 62 % [15].

Stone Size

Larger stones have a greater likelihood of retreatment, auxiliary procedures and complications with SWL than URS [16, 17].

Stone burden is commonly described via maximum stone diameter. Alternative methods, including stone area and volume have been demonstrated to be a predictors of treatment success as well [18]. Most recently, Bandi and colleagues performed a comparative analysis of several CT-based metrics of stone size [19]. They demonstrated that stone volume was a greater predictor of treatment success than stone diameter or area. It is felt that by including consideration of stone depth, stone volume renders more accurate characterization of the total burden.

Notably, most studies that include stone volume utilize specialized radiographic software and technicians to obtain these values. However, these resources are usually unavailable for most urologists. As such, it is important to note that stone volume can be calculated using the ellipsoid volume formula. This requires only manual measurement of stone height, width and depth ($volume = H \times W \times D \times \pi/6$). Tran et al. [20] recently demonstrated that this method yields a stone volume tightly correlated with the computer-generated values ($r = 0.9778$, in process).

Body Mass Index and Skin-to-Stone Distance

Patient body habitus has a significant impact on SWL efficiency. The energy of the shockwave diminishes by 10–20 % for every 6 cm of tissue it traverses [21]. Also, many lithotripters have a maximum focal point of approximately 12–14 cm [22].

Body mass index (BMI) is a readily available metric that is an established risk factor for SWL failure. Pareek et al. [23] showed a significant difference in BMI between stone-free patients and those with residual stones (BMI 26.9 ± 0.5 vs. BMI 30.8 ± 0.9, $p < 0.05$) [23]. A recent multivariate analysis by Hwang et al. [24] demonstrated that patients with BMI >25 had a 3.5 times greater risk of SWL failure [24]. Yang and colleagues [25] demonstrated similar results, with BMI and buttock circumference being noted as predictors of SWL failure [25].

Skin-to-Stone Distance (SSD) is another predictor related to body habitus. This metric attempts to measure the presumed path of the shockwave by averaging the horizontal, vertical and diagonal distance from the stone to the skin. It is theorized that by measuring the amount of soft tissue that a shockwave must traverse, SSD can provide a more precise assessment of the dampening forces than BMI. A cut-off value of 10 cm was noted by Pareek et al. [23] to be predictive of SWL failure for renal stones [26]. Similarly, Patel et al. [27] showed that SSD of 10.7 cm had a significantly greater residual stone rate compared with patients with SSD of 8.3 cm [27].

Combination Scores

Simultaneous consideration of these many CT-based metrics can be challenging. Metrics that allow for combined analysis of pre-operative factors can augment predictive power and allow for easier application of these tools in clinical practice.

Simultaneous consideration of two parameters has been utilized by Perks et al. [28] where stones <900 HU and SSD <9 cm correlated with SWL success, regardless of stone size, location of BMI [28].

Ng et al. [29] considered ureteral stones and determined cutoff values of 593 HU, 9.2 cm and 200 mL for stone density, SSD and volume, respectively [29]. They then utilized a scoring system where having 0, 1, 2 or 3 of these factors correlated with 17.9, 48.4, 73.3 and 100 % success rates.

Similarly, Tran et al. (2014) developed the Triple D (DDD) Score for prediction of SWL success for ureteral and renal stones. Recent analysis has demonstrated that SWL is more cost-effective than URS when its stone-free rate is greater than 65 % [30]. Therefore, these predictive tools, while still in the experimental stages, hold great promise for identifying the ideal candidates for SWL.

Intraoperative Tools to Improve Efficacy

In addition to identification of proper treatment candidates, SWL treatment success can be further optimized by utilization of ideal treatment strategies.

Lowering shockwave delivery rate (from 120 shocks per minute to 60) and power ramping (starting at low power and gradually increasing to full power) can improve stone fragmentation and limit renal injury [31, 32].

In addition, optimizing acoustic coupling can significantly improve treatment efficacy. Shockwaves pass efficiently through water, coupling gel and body tissue, but their propagation is significantly limited by air pockets. As little as 2 % air bubbles within the coupling medium can decrease stone fragmentation by 20–40 % [33]. Thus, while easily overlooked, proper application of coupling gel is an important consideration in the optimization of SWL.

Medical Expulsive Therapy and Shockwave Lithotripsy

Postoperative administration of tamsulosin has been demonstrated to improve SWL outcomes. Limiting ureteral spasm can promote more efficient passage of residual fragments. A meta-analysis of 15 randomized studies that included over 1,300 patients revealed a 24 % improvement in stone passage rates after SWL of ureteral and renal stones [34]. This benefit was even greater with proximal stones

(RR = 1.83, 95 % CI 1.20–2.78) and distal stones (RR = 1.43, 95 % CI 1.13–1.81). Similar to MET data for spontaneous passage, tamsulosin improved passage rates and also was associated with shorter time to stone passage and fewer pain episodes.

Newer Devices

Reports of the experience with newer generation lithotripters has generated optimism related to the high stone-free rates for the treatment of ureteral urolithiasis. These lithotripters deliver the shock wave energy over a larger surface area of patient skin, which helps to decrease pain. The importance of the lessened pain with these devices lies not only in potentially easier convalescence for the patient but also a decreased anesthetic requirement as SWL with these lithotripters is often readily performed with either intravenous sedation or minimal anesthesia.

In addition, the delivery of shockwaves is focused to a smaller focal area, which can facilitate more effective stone fragmentation. The more concentrated delivery of energy, however may lead to a greater risk of subcapsular hematoma formation in comparison to the first generation spark-gap lithotripters.

Ureteroscopy

Large instruments and poor optics initially made access to the upper ureter challenging. Therefore, URS was initially limited to treating stones in the distal and mid-ureter while proximal stones were treated with SWL. In addition, early intracorporeal lithotripsy options were inefficient. Thus, URS beyond the distal ureter was initially a harrowing task associated with a higher risk of complications.

Significant advancements in technology over the last two decades have made URS safer and more reliable. Miniaturization of instruments reduced the need for routine ureteral dilation and has contributed to the decreased rates of serious complications such as ureteral stricture formation or perforation. Perforation rates ranging between 2 and 4 % have been noted, with lower rates cited in modern series [35, 36].

While it requires general anesthesia, is more invasive, and is oftentimes completed with stent placement, URS does offer some advantages over SWL.

First, while SWL single-session stone-free rates can vary significantly, URS has been reported to have consistent stone-free rates of 85–100 % after a single treatment [35].

Also, while patient and stone-related factors have proven to affect SWL outcomes, there is a paucity of evidence that these parameters affect URS efficacy. Several studies have demonstrated no difference in stone-free rates or complications amongst overweight patients undergoing URS [37, 38]. In addition, while stones with greater density may require more time for fragmentation, the holmium laser has been proven to break stones of all compositions [39].

Lastly, URS is useful for specific patient populations that are poor candidates for SWL. While SWL is contraindicated for patients with bleeding diatheses and/or on anti-coagulation therapy, URS has no increased risk of significant bleeding in this population [40]. Also, treatment of multiple stones in multiple locations is challenging with SWL, however single-session clearance of these stones can be more readily attained with URS [41].

Factors that do appear to affect URS success rates are as follows:

Preoperative stent placement

Placement of stent prior to stone treatment yields passive ureteral dilation, allowing easier access to the upper tract. Netsch et al. [42] demonstrated in a matched-pair comparative analysis that when a stent was present prior to URS treatment, stone-free rates were 15 % greater (98.2 % vs 83.3 %, $p<0.01$) amongst patients with a larger stone burden (greater than 5 mm) [42].

Drawing from these findings, some have argued that this improvement justifies stent placement prior to stone treatment for larger stone burdens. While pre-stenting certainly allows for easier treatment, the guarantee of a second procedure raises concerns regarding the cost-effectiveness of this maneuver.

Stone burden

The total stone burden being targeted is a predictor of treatment success. Similar to SWL, new methods for accurate assessment of stone burden are being investigated. Stone volume is the most accurate predictor of stone-free status after URS. However, it takes more time to measure than maximum stone diameter. Ito et al. [43] reported that stone volume does not need to be calculated in cases where stone diameter is <20 mm, as it is no better at predicting outcome in these patients [43]. Surface area, while slightly inferior to stone volume, was also demonstrated to be an accurate predictor of stone-free status after URS [44, 45]. The advantage of using surface area is that it can be calculated from plain-film X-ray.

As mentioned above, *stone density* does not affect stone-free rates, but it does affect the efficiency of stone fragmentation. Using the holmium laser, Ito et al. [39] showed that stones measured to have higher HU require more time for fragmentation [39].

One of the chief disadvantages for URS is its greater frequency of stent placement compared with SWL. Stent-related lower urinary tract symptoms significantly worsen patient quality of life. Also, they often require a secondary procedure for removal and are associated with complications such as infection, encrustation and migration [45]. Several well-designed studies have confirmed that stenting after routine URS is not required [46]. The 2007 AUA/EUA Guideline on Management of Ureteral Calculi states, "stenting following uncomplicated URS is optional"[6]. However, stenting post-ureteroscopy appears to remain a common practice. A 2014 international multi-center prospective study that included nearly 10,000 patients treated between 2010 and 2012 revealed that 80.6 % of patients had postoperative stent placement [36].

Outcomes for Shockwave Lithotripsy, Ureteroscopy and Alternatives

Considerations

Accurate comparison of URS and SWL is difficult for two reasons. First, the technology is continually evolving. These changes can be dramatic and result in significant changes with stone-free rates (both positive and negative). Second, there is a relative scarcity of high-level evidence to assess the new technologies available in the modern era. Therefore, conclusions are often drawn from studies that are either less relevant or of lower quality.

To illustrate this challenge, consider that in 2001 a prospective, randomized controlled trial demonstrated equivalent stone-free rates for SWL and URS in treating distal ureteral stones [35]. However, SWL was performed with the Dornier HM3 lithotripter, which is no longer used and URS was performed with scopes and intracorporeal lithotripsy devices that are considered outdated today. Thus, despite a high level of evidence, the applicability of these results to the current practice environment is limited.

To enhance the utility of the information presented here, we will emphasize studies performed with equipment that is commonplace in this contemporary era.

Proximal Ureteral Stones

Direct Comparison Between Shockwave Lithotripsy and Ureteroscopy

Seven studies have provided direct comparison between treatment modalities for proximal stones (Table 4.1). Six compared SWL to URS. One study compared URS, PCNL and laparoscopic ureterolithotomy. However, only one of these studies compared third-generation lithotripters to URS with holmium laser – the current standards for this modern era.

In general, single-session treatment with ureteroscopy had much higher and more consistent stone-free rates (86.6–97.5 %) than SWL (35–77.5 %). Efficiency quotients (EQ) were significantly worse for SWL in three of five studies that included this measure. Complication rates tended to be higher for URS, however the overall incidence was low.

Amongst the studies that noted quality of life, the findings were variable. Patients with SWL presented more often to the ER and office with renal colic, whereas URS patients sought care more frequently for stent-related lower urinary tract symptoms.

Kumar et al. [47] compared semi-rigid URS with holmium laser to SWL with a third-generation lithotripter [47]. Mean stone size was 12.5 and 12.3 cm for URS and SWL patients, respectively. While no significant difference was noted in stone-free rates, a significantly higher re-treatment rate was required for SWL (61.1 % vs. 11.1 %, $p<0.0001$, average 1.6 SWL sessions). As expected, the EQ was higher for

Table 4.1 Treatment of proximal ureteral stones

Study (ref)	Year	F/U	Patients	SWL lithotriptor	URS/lithotripsy	Mean stone size	SFR URS	SFR SWL	Comp URS	Comp SWL
Lee et al. [73]	2006	NR	20 URS, 22 SWL	Siemen AG Lithostar 2	EHL/Lithoclast	18.5 mm (URS), 17.9 mm (SWL)	35 %	32 %	25 % uperf, 30 % fever	5 %
Salem [74]	2009	2 weeks–3 months	200	HM3	Semirigid URS/ Lithoclast	<20 mm			17 %	29 %
>10 mm						12.2 mm (URS), 12.5 mm (SWL)	88 %	60 %		
<10 mm						6.8 mm (URS), 6.2 mm (SWL)	100 %	80 %		
Kumar et al. [47] (overall results)	2013	3 months	180	Dornier Compact Delta	Semirigid URS/ Holmium	12.5 mm (URS), 12.3 mm (SWL)	87 %	82 %	11 %	6.6 %
<10 mm							88 %	85 %		
10–20 mm							85 %	78 %		
Cui et al. [48]	2014	3–6 months	80 URS, 80 SWL	3rd Gen Dornier	Semirigid URS/ Holmium	10.2 mm (URS), 9.8 mm (SWL)	98 %	78 %	0 %	0 %
Parker et al. [75] (Overall results)	2004	6 months	109 URS, 111 SWL	2nd Gen HM4 or DoLi-S	Flexible and Semirigid URS/ Holmium		91 %[a]	55 %[a]		
<10 mm							90 %[a]	60 %[a]	6.2 %	2.7 %
>10 mm							93 %[a]	45 %[a]	7.1 %	0 %
Basiri et al. [49]	2008	3 weeks	50 URS, 50 Lap, 50 PCNL		Semirigid URS/ Pneumatic and Laser	17.8 mm URS, 22.4 mm Lap, 20.3 mm PCNL	76 % URS, 90 % Lap, 86 % PCNL		0 % URS, 16 % Lap, 18 % PCNL	

(continued)

Table 4.1 (continued)

Study (ref)	Year	F/U	Patients	SWL lithotriptor	URS/lithotripsy	Mean stone size	SFR URS	SFR SWL	Comp URS	Comp SWL
Wu et al. [76]	2004	4 weeks	39 URS, 41 SWL	Medispec Econolith 2000	Semirigid URS, Holmium	15.1 mm URS, 12.8 SWL[a]	88[a]	61 %[a]	0 % uperf, 0 % hemat	
Sun et al. [50]	2008	4 weeks	43 Ant URS, 44 Ret URS		Ant : Semirigid, Ret: Flexible URS, Both w/Holmium Laser	14.6 mm Ant, 14.7 mm Ret	100 %[a] Ret, 86 % Ant[a]		1/43 severe bleed; 1/44 uperf	

Ref reference number, *F/U* follow-up, *mo* months, *wks* weeks, *NR* not reported, *URS* ureteroscopy, *SWL* shock wave lithotripsy, *Lap* laparoscopic ureterolithotomy, *PCNL* percutaneous nephrolithotomy, *SFR* stone free rate, *Ant* antegrade ureteroscopy, *Ret* retrograde ureteroscopy, *Aux* rate of auxillary procedures, *Mean Ses* mean number of SWL sessions, *Comp* complication rate

[a]Statistically significant difference between parameters measured between URS and SWL, *uperf* ureteral perforation, *hemat* renal hematoma

URS, especially for stones larger than 10 mm (83.4 vs 46.4, p=0.01). The overall complication rate was higher for URS (11.1 % vs. 6.6 %), but this difference was not statistically significant. There was no difference in the incidence of UTI or severe pain amongst the two groups.

Although a retrospective analysis, Cui et al. [48] provide an interesting comparison between SWL with a third-generation device and URS with holmium laser [48]. Mean stone size was approximately 10 mm for each group. Stone-free rates were ultimately similar (92.5 % SWL vs. 97.5 % URS) although single session SFR for SWL was 77.5 %. URS patients had significantly more lower urinary tract symptoms. URS costs were greater, largely because of its average 2-day hospitalization. Patient satisfaction scores were similar for the two modalities.

Percutaneous antegrade ureteroscopy is an alternative approach for proximal ureteral stones. Basiri et al. [49] randomized 150 patients to URS, PCNL or laparoscopic ureterolithotomy [49]. There was no significant difference in stone-free rates between URS and PCNL (76 % vs. 86 %, p=0.2). Eighteen percent of patients that had PCNL had persistent urinary leak >3 days beyond surgery. The stone-free rate for the laparoscopic approach was 90 %, however two patients required conversion to open surgery and eight patients (18 %) had a persistent urinary leakage.

Sun et al. [50] compared retrograde URS with "mini" percutaneous antegrade ureteroscopy for impacted proximal stones [50]. Antegrade URS was performed with an 8Fr or 9.5Fr semi-rigid scope through a small access channel. The average stone size was 14.6 mm. A higher stone-free rate was noted for the antegrade approach (100 % vs 86.4 %, p=0.02), however operative times, hospital stay, and return to normal activities was significantly greater for this group. Minimally-invasive methods to perform antegrade stone treatment for this challenging patient population continue to be investigated [51, 52].

Matlaga et al. conducted a systematic review in 2012 of randomized controlled trials [53]. This study deliberately separated studies that utilized the HM3 lithotripter and subsequent generation devices due to the noted differences in results [54]. Relevant findings for proximal stones included a greater probability of being stone free with URS than SWL with HM3 (RR 1.35) and other lithotripters (RR 1.15). The chance of re-treatment, notably, was much higher with HM3 and other SWL devices (RR 0.14 and RR 0.08, respectively, compared with URS). URS had a higher likelihood of complications than either SWL modality.

Shockwave Lithotripsy for Proximal Ureteral Stones

Consideration of the performance of the new third-generation lithotripters may help to provide a clearer understanding of the current state of modern SWL. As noted above, the Dornier HM3 delivered consistently high stone-free rates. Second generation devices offered improved portability and decreased anesthetic requirements but sacrificed treatment efficacy. Third-generation devices have been associated with an overall improvement in outcomes while maintaining the decreased anesthetic requirement and faster convalescence.

Neisius et al. [55] evaluated the Siemens Lithoskop device for ureteral and renal stones [55]. Amongst stones less than 10 mm, the overall success rate was 95 % after an average of 1.3 treatment sessions. When all treated stones were considered (size range 4–25 mm), a 93 % stone free rate after an average of 1.4 sessions was reported. Nearly 80 % of patients were stone free after a single treatment.

These results are in keeping with those reported in other studies of third-generation devices over the last half-decade (Table 4.2). Stone-free rates for proximal stones ranged from 85 to 97 %. Treatment sessions required ranged from 1.2 to 1.4. It should be noted those studies that reported higher retreatment rates featured more aggressive thresholds for re-treatment (i.e. treating all residual fragments >4 mm) in comparison to studies that followed a more conservative approach (i.e. trial of passage for stones <5 mm). Importantly, these studies reported mean stone burden less than 10 mm.

These findings indicate that in a properly selected population, SWL for proximal stones with third-generation lithotripters yields good treatment success rates (Table 4.3).

Ureteroscopy for Proximal Ureteral Stones

Consideration of recent studies with URS and holmium laser demonstrate consistently excellent treatment success rates.

Perez Castro et al. [36] reported of an international multi-center prospective study evaluating the outcomes of URS on nearly 10,000 patients between 2010 and 2012. This large data set, which acquired information from low and high volume centers as well as community and teaching hospitals, provides perhaps the most representative depiction of todays' treatment landscape. Notable findings from this study included an overall stone free rate of 84.5 % for proximal stones (n=2,656).

Approximately eighty percent (80.6 %) of patients had postoperative stents placed following ureteroscopy. Ureteral perforation (0.7–1.6 % depending on stone location) was the most common significant intraoperative complication and ureteral avulsion was a rare event (0.1–0.3 %). Postoperatively, fever was the most common complication (1.3–1.5 %), followed by UTI (0.6–1.0 %), while the incidence of sepsis was rare (0.1–0.5 %).

Mid-ureteral Stones

The mid-ureter is traditionally defined with borders between the upper and lower border of the sacrum. The prominence of pelvic bone in this location makes localization of calculi during SWL challenging. No randomized trials were identified that compared treatment modalities for stones in the mid-ureter.

Overview of recent reports for SWL and URS indicate that both modalities are able to achieve good stone-free rates. Recent studies of third generation lithotripters

Table 4.2 Treatment of distal ureteral stones

Study (ref)	Year	F/U	Patients	SWL lithotriptor	URS/lithotripsy	Mean stone size (mm)	SFR URS (%)	SFR SWL (%)	Comp URS (%)	Comp SWL (%)
Verze et al. [77]	2010	3 months	137 SWL, 136 URS	Modulith SLX	Semirigid URS/ EHL and Lithoclast	10 (SWL), 10 (URS)	95	92.7	19	15
Pearle et al. [35]	2001	3 months	32 SWL, 32 URS	Dornier HM3	Semirigid URS/Ho: YAG	7.4 (URS), 6.4 (SWL)	100	100	25	9
Hendrikx et al. [78]	1999	3 months	69 SWL, 87 URS	Dornier HM4	Semirigid URS/ Pulse-dye laser and EHL	>5	91[a]	51[a]	25[a]	4[a]
Peschel et al. [79]	1999	6 weeks	40 SWL, 40 URS	Dornier MFL 5,000	Semirigid URS/ Lithoclast	9.6 (SWL), 8.9 (URS)	100	95	0	0
						3.9 (SWL), 4.0 (URS)	100	85	0	0

Ref reference number, *Prox* proximal, *F/U* follow-up, *mo* months, *SFR* stone free rate, *Aux* rate of auxillary procedures, *Mean Ses* mean number of SWL sessions, *Comp* complication rate for SWL, *EQ* efficiency quotient, *STI* stone treatment index

[a]Statistically significant difference between URS and SWL group in parameter being measured

Table 4.3 Third generation lithotriptors

Study (ref)	Year	Location	F/U	Patients	SWL lithotriptor	Stone size [stone area]	SFR SWL (%)	Aux (%)	Mean Ses	Comp (%)	EQ SWL
Egilmez et al. [80]	2007	Prox	3 months	483	Lithostar Modularis Uro-Plus (Siemens)	[92 mm^2]	86	7	1.2	1	0.71
		Mid					86				0.66
		Distal					85				0.67
De Sio et al. [81]	2007	Prox	3 months	63	Modulith-SLX-F2 (Storz)	9.5 mm (5–15)	92	6.3	1.2	3.8	0.63
		Distal					76				
Murota-Kawano et al. [82]	2008	Prox	3 months	401	Compact Delta (Dornier)	9.9 mm	92.6	2	1.2	0.2	
		Mid/distal					97.6				
Tiselius [83]	2008	Prox	2 months	254	Modulith SLX Classic (Storz)	[53 mm^2]	73.1	18	1.37		STI 5.3
		Mid		90		[47 mm^2]	66.7		1.47		STI 4.59
		Distal		236		[38 mm^2]	83.2		1.22		STI 5.15
Seitz et al. [84]	2008	Prox	3 months	26	Lithoskop (Siemens)	8 mm (4–20)	85	18	2	3.7	0.61–0.73
		Mid		33			82		1.4		
		Distal		31			97		1.2		
Neisius et al. [55]	2013	Prox	3 months	99	Lithoskop (Siemens)	8 mm (4–28)	93	7.1	1.3	0.5	0.68
		Mid					90				0.68
		Distal					94				0.73

Ref reference number, *Prox* proximal, *F/U* follow-up, *mo* months, *SFR* stone free rate, *Aux* rate of auxillary procedures, *Mean Ses* mean number of SWL sessions, *Comp* complication rate for SWL, *EQ* efficiency quotient, *STI* stone treatment index for the treatment of mid-ureteral stones revealed stone-free rates between 82 and 100 %. Notably, these series were conducted primarily on smaller stones ranging in size between 8 and 10 mm. The mean number of treatments ranged from 1.3 to nearly 1.5.

In a recent large, multicenter report, treatment of mid-ureteral stones had an 89.4 % overall success rate [36]. Interestingly, treatment of these stones was associated with the greatest incidence of ureteral perforation (1.6 %) compared to stones in other locations. Perhaps contributing to this higher complication rate was that 64 % of these patients had impacted stones.

Distal Ureteral Stones

Comparison Between Shockwave Lithotripsy and Ureteroscopy

A total of five randomized-controlled trials were identified that compared URS to SWL for distal ureterolithiasis. The most recent of these provided a prospective comparison between a third-generation lithotripter and URS with holmium laser. In this study, Verze et al. (2010) randomized 273 patients to SWL or URS. [56] Mean stone size was 10 cm. Overall stone-free rates were similar (SWL 92.7 % vs. URS 94.8 %) however the re-treatment rate for SWL was significantly higher (44.8 % vs. 7.8 %, $p<0.05$). In comparison to smaller stones, patients with stones greater than 1 cm had a higher SWL re-treatment rate (80.3 % vs. 12.1 %), need for auxiliary procedures (19.7 % vs. 3.0 %) and complication rate (27.9 % vs. 7.2 %). These findings suggest SWL for distal stones <1 cm is a good option but URS is better for stones >1 cm.

Matlaga et al. compared the five randomized controlled trials in a meta-analysis [53]. Their findings indicated that following a single treatment, URS had similar stone-free rates to SWL with the HM3 lithotripter, however, when SWL was performed with non-HM3 devices, URS had significantly higher success rates (RR 1.55, 95 % CI 1.13–2.56). In addition, patients treated with URS were nearly seven-times less likely to require re-treatment (RR 0.14). Complication rates were nearly 30 % higher with URS but this value was not statistically significant. It is important to keep in mind that these findings are derived from four studies from 1999 to 2002 and one from 2010. Therefore, the applicability of the findings may be limited in the modern day.

Shockwave Lithotripsy for Distal Stones

Specific analysis of third-generation devices over the last 5 years demonstrate a stone-free rate ranging from 85 to 98 % with fewer treatment sessions needed in comparison to proximal and mid-ureteral stones (1.2–1.22). These studies are limited to stones less than 10 mm and, taken together, suggest that SWL can be an effective treatment option for smaller distal ureteral stones.

In women of childbearing age, SWL is typically not considered a treatment option for distal stones due to the theoretical risk of damage to the female reproductive tract and ovaries. Although no demonstrated effect on fertility has been reported, most centers either avoid use of SWL in this population or ensure that detailed consent is obtained from these patients prior to the procedure [57, 58].

Ureteroscopy for Distal Stones

As has been mentioned above, the advancements in technology for URS have allowed for a more consistent and safer procedure. Elashry et al. [59] demonstrated this in their report of 5,133 URS procedures where they compared results from patients treated between 1991 and 1995 to those treated thereafter. Intraoperative and postoperative complication rates were significantly lower, (4.1 % vs. 15.1 % and 8 % vs. 16.1 %, respectively, $p<0.001$) and stone-free rates were over 10 % better (97.3 % vs. 85.7 %, $p<0.001$) for those treated in the later group [59].

The Perez Castro et al. [60] international multi-center prospective study demonstrated a similarly high stone-free rate of 94.2 % for distal stones ($n=4{,}479$). Ureteral perforation (0.7–1.6 % depending on stone location) was the most common significant intraoperative complication and avulsion a rare event (0.1–0.3 %). Postoperatively, fever was the most common complication (1.3–1.5 %), followed by UTI (0.6–1.0 %), while the incidence of sepsis was rare (0.1–0.5 %) [60].

Special Considerations

Pregnancy

Symptomatic ureterolithiasis is the most common non-obstetric reason for hospitalization during pregnancy. The incidence is reported to be as high as 1 in 200 pregnancies [61]. There is an increased risk of stone formation in these patients due to increased renal handling of calcium, salt and uric acid [62]. Placental production of vitamin D further enhances the hypercalciuria of pregnancy. Lastly, hormone-mediated dilation of collecting system during pregnancy is hypothesized to facilitate migration of renal stones into ureter [63].

Acute stone episodes pose a risk for the pregnant patient. The stress of the event elevates the risk of pre-term labor, premature rupture of membranes and preterm delivery [64]. While 70–80 % of women will experience spontaneous stone passage, 20–30 % require intervention.

Urinary tract decompression without stone treatment is the traditionally espoused course of action for women that require intervention [6]. Yet the altered physicochemistry of urine during pregnancy can precipitate rapid stent encrustation, thereby requiring exchange nearly every 4–6 weeks. Indwelling stents also facilitate the development of bacteriuria and urinary tract infection. In light of these concerns, it is important to consider stone treatment in appropriately selected patients.

SWL is not a feasible option during pregnancy due to the risk of harming the fetus with fluoroscopy and shockwaves. URS, however, is safe and effective in this population. The holmium laser minimizes tissue penetration, limiting the risk of injury to the fetus. Combined spinal and local anesthesia has also been reported to be successful in recent reported studies.

Laing et al. [61] reviewed the last ten years of URS stone treatment in pregnant women [61]. A total of 116 patients from 15 studies were considered in their analyses. The combined treatment success rate was 86 %. Complications were rare, with a low rate of UTI (4 %) and a very low rate of severe complications such as ureteral perforation and premature uterine contractions (0.8 % each).

Safe URS with minimizing anesthesia appears to be achievable in this population as well. 23.4 % (23/98) of patients received general anesthesia, while the other 75 patients (76.5 %) received only local and/or spinal anesthesia. No anesthetic complications were reported.

While it is important to consider the possibility of publication bias limiting the publication of studies with unfavorable results, based upon the available literature, it appears that URS can be a safe and effective treatment option for pregnant women with stones.

Alterations in urinary composition and urinary tract anatomy facilitate stone formation and passage in pregnant women. The standard of care for treatment of symptomatic ureterolithiasis in pregnant women is urinary tract decompression, however frequent stent exchange due to rapid encrustation is common. URS is a viable treatment option for these patients and can be performed safely with minimal anesthesia.

Pediatrics

Ureteral stones in pediatric patients present a unique challenge.

To begin, accurate characterization of stone burden and location is often limited due to concerns about radiation exposure. Ultrasound and plain film x-ray are the typical imaging studies obtained. While ultrasound features a high sensitivity for detection of hydronephrosis and renal stones, its sensitivity for identifying ureteral stones is only 45 % [65]. Ultrasound also often overestimates stone size, especially for stones less than 5 mm.

Plain film x-ray provides more accurate information on stone size and location, however radio-opaque calculi are only identified in approximately 40–60 % of cases [66].

Given this, urologists can encounter significant uncertainty in the management of these patients. While computed tomography imaging offers greater sensitivity and specificity for detection of ureterolithiasis, there is hesitancy to obtain this due to radiation risk. However, several recent studies characterize the risks of CT to be minimal in comparison to the benefit [67]. Thus, when clinically indicated, CT scan should be obtained.

When deciding whether to allow a trial of passage, it is important to consider that children have a narrower ureter than adults. Thus, in comparison to the typical threshold of 5 mm for adults, the likelihood of stone passage is significant lower amongst stones less than 5 mm [68].

Medical expulsive therapy is an important therapeutic adjunct in pediatric patients. A randomized study that compared 30 children taking tamsulosin to 30 children taking placebo reported a significant improvement in passage rate (88 % vs 64 %) and time to stone passage (8.2 vs 14.5 days) [69]. Less pain and need for analgesics was noted. No significant adverse effects were reported.

SWL stone free rates have, in general, been higher for children than adults, with success rates ranging from 80 to 95 % after an average of 1.5 treatment sessions [70]. This higher success rate is attributed to two factors. First, children are generally thinner than adults and therefore have a shorter distance through which shock-wave energy can be attenuated. In addition, children are also better able to pass residual stone fragments. This is believed to be due to increased ureteral elasticity and distensibility. The long-term consequences of SWL in children are uncertain.

While SWL was adopted early on in children, the use of URS was limited. Large instruments and limited experience raised concerns about ureteral injury and vesicoureteral reflux. However, miniaturization of ureteroscopes and the overall improvement in technology has allowed for greater experience with URS. High treatment success rates, ranging between 85 and 100 % for distal stones and 88–100 % for proximal stones have been reported [70]. Also, in comparison to single-session SWL, one randomized study noted a significantly higher SFR with URS (94 % vs 43 %) [71]. In addition, low rates of stricture and vesicoureteral reflux have been reported (0–1.7 % and 0–8 %, respectively), helping to allay initial concerns. Importantly, all reported cases of VUR were grade 1 and resolved spontaneously [72].

Take Home Points

- The likelihood of spontaneous passage of ureteral stones is high with stones <3 mm in size
- Medical expulsive therapy improves the likelihood of stone passage and increases stone passage rates.
- SWL is especially effective in the pediatric population, which has the advantage of greater ability to pass residual fragments and generally a leaner body habitus compared to adults.
- URS has a high single-session success rate. The incidence of ureteral injury or other major complications are low, with the utilization of small instruments and adjunctive devices available today.

References

1. Scales Jr CD, Smith AC, Hanley JM, Saigal CS. Urologic diseases in America P. Prevalence of kidney stones in the United States. Eur Urol. 2012;62(1):160–5.
2. Teichman JM. Clinical practice. Acute renal colic from ureteral calculus. N Engl J Med. 2004;350(7):684–93.
3. Matlaga BR. American board of U. Contemporary surgical management of upper urinary tract calculi. J Urol. 2009;181(5):2152–6.

4. Tiselius HG. Removal of ureteral stones with extracorporeal shock wave lithotripsy and ureteroscopic procedures. What can we learn from the literature in terms of results and treatment efforts? Urol Res. 2005;33(3):185–90.
5. Gerber GS, Acharya SS. Management of ureteral calculi. J Endourol. 2010;24(6):953–4.
6. Preminger GM, Tiselius HG, Assimos DG, et al. 2007 guideline for the management of ureteral calculi. J Urol. 2007;178(6):2418–34.
7. Sivula A, Lehtonen T. Spontaneous passage of artificial concretions applied in the rabbit ureter. Scand J Urol Nephrol. 1967;1(3):259–63.
8. Hollingsworth JM, Rogers MA, Kaufman SR, et al. Medical therapy to facilitate urinary stone passage: a meta-analysis. Lancet. 2006;368(9542):1171–9.
9. Campschroer T, Zhu Y, Duijvesz D, Grobbee DE, Lock MT. Alpha-blockers as medical expulsive therapy for ureteral stones. Cochrane Database Syst Rev. 2014;(4):CD008509.
10. Hollingsworth JM, Wolf Jr JS, Faerber GJ, Roberts WW, Dunn RL, Hollenbeck BK. Understanding the barriers to the dissemination of medical expulsive therapy. J Urol. 2010; 184(6):2368–72.
11. Klee LW, Brito CG, Lingeman JE. The clinical implications of brushite calculi. J Urol. 1991;145(4):715–8.
12. Kim SC, Burns EK, Lingeman JE, Paterson RF, McAteer JA, Williams Jr JC. Cystine calculi: correlation of CT-visible structure, CT number, and stone morphology with fragmentation by shock wave lithotripsy. Urol Res. 2007;35(6):319–24.
13. Wang LJ, Wong YC, Chuang CK, et al. Predictions of outcomes of renal stones after extracorporeal shock wave lithotripsy from stone characteristics determined by unenhanced helical computed tomography: a multivariate analysis. Eur Radiol. 2005;15(11):2238–43.
14. el Assmy A, Abou-el-Ghar ME, el Nahas AR, Refaie HF, Sheir KZ. Multidetector computed tomography: role in determination of urinary stones composition and disintegration with extracorporeal shock wave lithotrips an in vitro study. Urology. 2011;77(2):286–90.
15. Ouzaid I, Al-qahtani S, Dominique S, et al. A 970 Hounsfield units (HU) threshold of kidney stone density on non-contrast computed tomography (NCCT) improves patients' selection for extracorporeal shockwave lithotripsy (ESWL): evidence from a prospective study. BJU Int. 2012;110(11 Pt B):E438–42.
16. Nabi G, Baldo O, Cartledge J, Cross W, Joyce AD, Lloyd SN. The impact of the Dornier Compact Delta lithotriptor on the management of primary ureteric calculi. Eur Urol. 2003; 44(4):482–6.
17. Kijvikai K, Haleblian GE, Preminger GM, de la Rosette J. Shock wave lithotripsy or ureteroscopy for the management of proximal ureteral calculi: an old discussion revisited. J Urol. 2007;178(4 Pt 1):1157–63.
18. Buchholz NP, Rhabar MH, Talati J. Is measurement of stone surface area necessary for SWL treatment of nonstaghorn calculi? J Endourol. 2002;16(4):215–20.
19. Bandi G, Meiners RJ, Pickhardt PJ, Nakada SY. Stone measurement by volumetric three-dimensional computed tomography for predicting the outcome after extracorporeal shock wave lithotripsy. BJU Int. 2009;103(4):524–8.
20. Tran TY, McGillen K, Cone EB, Pareek G. Triple D Score is a Reportable Predictor of Shockwave Lithotripsy Stone-Free Rates. J Endourol 2014; epub Sept 19, 2014.
21. Jayanthi VR, Arnold PM, Koff SA. Strategies for managing upper tract calculi in young children. J Urol. 1999;162(3 Pt 2):1234–7.
22. Calvert RC, Burgess NA. Urolithiasis and obesity: metabolic and technical considerations. Curr Op Urol. 2005;15(2):113–7.
23. Pareek G, Armenakas NA, Panagopoulos G, Bruno JJ, Fracchia JA. Extracorporeal shock wave lithotripsy success based on body mass index and Hounsfield units. Urology. 2005;65(1): 33–6.
24. Hwang I, Jung SI, Kim KH, et al. Factors influencing the failure of extracorporeal shock wave lithotripsy with Piezolith 3000 in the management of solitary ureteral stone. Urolithiasis. 2014;42(3);263–7.
25. Yang TK, Yang HJ, Lee LM, Liao CH. Body mass index and buttock circumference are independent predictors of disintegration failure in extracorporeal shock wave lithotripsy for ureteral calculi. J Formos Med Assoc [Taiwan yi zhi]. 2013;112(7):421–5.

26. Pareek G, Hedican SP, Lee Jr FT, Nakada SY. Shock wave lithotripsy success determined by skin-to-stone distance on computed tomography. Urology. 2005;66(5):941–4.
27. Patel T, Kozakowski K, Hruby G, Gupta M. Skin to stone distance is an independent predictor of stone-free status following shockwave lithotripsy. J Endourol. 2009;23(9):1383–5.
28. Perks AE, Schuler TD, Lee J, et al. Stone attenuation and skin-to-stone distance on computed tomography predicts for stone fragmentation by shock wave lithotripsy. Urology. 2008;72(4): 765–9.
29. Ng CF, Siu DY, Wong A, Goggins W, Chan ES, Wong KT. Development of a scoring system from noncontrast computerized tomography measurements to improve the selection of upper ureteral stone for extracorporeal shock wave lithotripsy. J Urol. 2009;181(3):1151–7.
30. Cone EB, Eisner BH, Ursiny M, Pareek G. Cost-effectiveness comparison of renal calculi treated with ureteroscopic laser lithotripsy versus shockwave lithotripsy. J Endourol. 2014; 28(6):639–43.
31. Handa RK, McAteer JA, Connors BA, Liu Z, Lingeman JE, Evan AP. Optimising an escalating shockwave amplitude treatment strategy to protect the kidney from injury during shockwave lithotripsy. BJU Int. 2012;110(11 Pt C):E1041–7.
32. Semins MJ, Trock BJ, Matlaga BR. The effect of shock wave rate on the outcome of shock wave lithotripsy: a meta-analysis. J Urol. 2008;179(1):194–7; discussion 197.
33. Pishchalnikov YA, Neucks JS, VonDerHaar RJ, Pishchalnikova IV, Williams Jr JC, McAteer JA. Air pockets trapped during routine coupling in dry head lithotripsy can significantly decrease the delivery of shock wave energy. J Urol. 2006;176(6 Pt 1):2706–10.
34. Zheng S, Liu LR, Yuan HC, Wei Q. Tamsulosin as adjunctive treatment after shockwave lithotripsy in patients with upper urinary tract stones: a systematic review and meta-analysis. Scand J Urol Nephrol. 2010;44(6):425–32.
35. Pearle MS, Nadler R, Bercowsky E, et al. Prospective randomized trial comparing shock wave lithotripsy and ureteroscopy for management of distal ureteral calculi. J Urol. 2001;166(4): 1255–60.
36. Perez Castro E, Osther PJ, Jinga V, et al. Differences in ureteroscopic stone treatment and outcomes for distal, mid-, proximal, or multiple ureteral locations: the clinical research office of the endourological society ureteroscopy global study. Eur Urol. 2014;66(1):102–9.
37. Chew BH, Zavaglia B, Paterson RF, et al. A multicenter comparison of the safety and effectiveness of ureteroscopic laser lithotripsy in obese and normal weight patients. J Endourol. 2013;27(6):710–4.
38. Dash A, Schuster TG, Hollenbeck BK, Faerber GJ, Wolf Jr JS. Ureteroscopic treatment of renal calculi in morbidly obese patients: a stone-matched comparison. Urology. 2002;60(3): 393–7; discussion 397.
39. Ito H, Kawahara T, Terao H, et al. Predictive value of attenuation coefficients measured as Hounsfield units on noncontrast computed tomography during flexible ureteroscopy with holmium laser lithotripsy: a single-center experience. J Endoruol. 2012;26(9):1125–30.
40. Watterson JD, Girvan AR, Cook AJ, et al. Safety and efficacy of holmium: YAG laser lithotripsy in patients with bleeding diatheses. J Urol. 2002;168(2):442–5.
41. Bilgasem S, Pace KT, Dyer S, Honey RJ. Removal of asymptomatic ipsilateral renal stones following rigid ureteroscopy for ureteral stones. J Endourol. 2003;17(6):397–400.
42. Netsch C, Knipper S, Bach T, Herrmann TR, Gross AJ. Impact of preoperative ureteral stenting on stone-free rates of ureteroscopy for nephroureterolithiasis: a matched-paired analysis of 286 patients. Urology. 2012;80(6):1214–9.
43. Ito H, Kawahara T, Terao H, et al. Utility and limitation of cumulative stone diameter in predicting urinary stone burden at flexible ureteroscopy with holmium laser lithotripsy: a single-center experience. PLoS ONE. 2013;8(6):e65060.
44. Ito H, Kawahara T, Terao H, et al. Evaluation of preoperative measurement of stone surface area as a predictor of stone-free status after combined ureteroscopy with holmium laser lithotripsy: a single-center experience. J Endourol. 2013;27(6):715–21.

45. Borboroglu PG, Amling CL, Schenkman NS, et al. Ureteral stenting after ureteroscopy for distal ureteral calculi: a multi-institutional prospective randomized controlled study assessing pain, outcomes and complications. J Urol. 2001;166(5):1651–7.
46. Cheung MC, Lee F, Leung YL, Wong BB, Tam PC. A prospective randomized controlled trial on ureteral stenting after ureteroscopic holmium laser lithotripsy. J Urol. 2003;169(4): 1257–60.
47. Kumar A, Nanda B, Kumar N, Kumar R, Vasudeva P, Mohanty NK. A prospective randomized comparison between shockwave lithotripsy and semirigid ureteroscopy for upper ureteral stones <2 cm: a single center experience. J Endourol. Epub Sep 12 2013.
48. Cui Y, Cao W, Shen H, et al. Comparison of ESWL and ureteroscopic holmium laser lithotripsy in management of ureteral stones. PLoS ONE. 2014;9(2):e87634.
49. Basiri A, Simforoosh N, Ziaee A, Shayaninasab H, Moghaddam SM, Zare S. Retrograde, antegrade, and laparoscopic approaches for the management of large, proximal ureteral stones: a randomized clinical trial. J Endourol. 2008;22(12):2677–80.
50. Sun X, Xia S, Lu J, Liu H, Han B, Li W. Treatment of large impacted proximal ureteral stones: randomized comparison of percutaneous antegrade ureterolithotripsy versus retrograde ureterolithotripsy. J Endourol. 2008;22(5):913–7.
51. Aravantinos E, Anagnostou T, Samarinas M, et al. Two-step minipercutaneous ureterolithotripsy under multimodal analgesia for complicated impacted calculi in proximal ureter. Urology. 2013;81(6):1147–52.
52. Moufid K, Abbaka N, Touiti D, Adermouch L, Amine M, Lezrek M. Large impacted upper ureteral calculi: a comparative study between retrograde ureterolithotripsy and percutaneous antegrade ureterolithotripsy in the modified lateral position. Urol Ann. 2013;5(3):140–6.
53. Matlaga BR, Jansen JP, Meckley LM, Byrne TW, Lingeman JE. Treatment of ureteral and renal stones: a systematic review and meta-analysis of randomized, controlled trials. J Urol. 2012;188(1):130–7.
54. Zehnder P, Roth B, Birkhauser F, et al. A prospective randomised trial comparing the modified HM3 with the MODULITH (R) SLX-F2 lithotripter. Eur Urol. 2011;59(4):637–44.
55. Neisius A, Wollner J, Thomas C, et al. Treatment efficacy and outcomes using a third generation shockwave lithotripter. BJU Int. 2013;112(7):972–81.
56. Verze P, Imbimbo C, Cancelmo G, et al. Extracorporeal shockwave lithotripsy vs ureteroscopy as first-line therapy for patients with single, distal ureteric stones: a prospective randomized study. BJU Int. 2010;106(11):1748–52.
57. Vieweg J, Weber HM, Miller K, Hautmann R. Female fertility following extracorporeal shock wave lithotripsy of distal ureteral calculi. J Urol. 1992;148(3 Pt 2):1007–10.
58. Erturk E, Ptak AM, Monaghan J. Fertility measures in women after extracorporeal shockwave lithotripsy of distal ureteral stones. J Endourol. 1997;11(5):315–7.
59. Elashry OM, Elgamasy AK, Sabaa MA, Abo-Elenien M, Omar MA, Eltataway HH, El-Abd SA. Ureteroscopic management of lower ureteric calculi: a 15-year single-centre experience. BJU Int. 2008;102(8):1010–7.
60. Perez Castro E, Osther PJ, Jinga V, Razvi H, Stravodimos KG, Parikh K, Kural AR, de la Rosette JJ. CROES Ureteroscopy Global Study Group. Differences in ureteroscopic stone treatment and outcomes for distal, mid-, proximal, or multiple ureteral locations: the clinical research office of the endourological society ureteroscopy global study. Eur Urol. 2014;66(1):102–9.
61. Gorton E, Whitfield HN. Renal calculi in pregnancy. Br J Urol. 1997;80 Suppl 1:4–9.
62. McAleer SJ, Loughlin KR. Nephrolithiasis and pregnancy. Curr Op Urol. 2004;14(2):123–7.
63. Laing KA, Lam TB, McClinton S, Cohen NP, Traxer O, Somani BK. Outcomes of ureteroscopy for stone disease in pregnancy: results from a systematic review of the literature. Urol Int. 2012;89(4):380–6.
64. Swartz MA, Lydon-Rochelle MT, Simon D, Wright JL, Porter MP. Admission for nephrolithiasis in pregnancy and risk of adverse birth outcomes. Obstet Gynecol. 2007;109(5): 1099–104.

65. Ray AA, Ghiculete D, Pace KT, Honey RJ. Limitations to ultrasound in the detection and measurement of urinary tract calculi. Urology. 2010;76(2):295–300.
66. Mitterberger M, Pinggera GM, Pallwein L, et al. Plain abdominal radiography with transabdominal native tissue harmonic imaging ultrasonography vs unenhanced computed tomography in renal colic. BJU Int. 2007;100(4):887–90.
67. Brody AS, Frush DP, Huda W, Brent RL. American Academy of Pediatrics Section on R. Radiation risk to children from computed tomography. Pediatrics. 2007;120(3):677–82.
68. Van Savage JG, Palanca LG, Andersen RD, Rao GS, Slaughenhoupt BL. Treatment of distal ureteral stones in children: similarities to the american urological association guidelines in adults. J Urol. 2000;164(3 Pt 2):1089–93.
69. Mokhless I, Zahran AR, Youssif M, Fahmy A. Tamsulosin for the management of distal ureteral stones in children: a prospective randomized study. J Ped Urol. 2012;8(5):544–8.
70. Smaldone MC, Corcoran AT, Docimo SG, Ost MC. Endourological management of pediatric stone disease: present status. J Urol. 2009;181(1):17–28.
71. De Dominicis M, Matarazzo E, Capozza N, Collura G, Caione P. Retrograde ureteroscopy for distal ureteric stone removal in children. BJU Int. 2005;95(7):1049–52.
72. Smaldone MC, Cannon Jr GM, Wu HY, et al. Is ureteroscopy first line treatment for pediatric stone disease? J Urol. 2007;178(5):2128–31; discussion 2131.
73. Lee YH, Tsai JY, Jiaan BP, Wu T, Yu CC. Prospective randomized trial comparing shock wave lithotripsy and ureteroscopic lithotripsy for management of large upper third ureteral stones. Urology. 2006;67(3):480–4; discussion 484.
74. Salem HK. A prospective randomized study comparing shock wave lithotripsy and semirigid ureteroscopy for the management of proximal ureteral calculi. Urology. 2009;74(6):1216–21.
75. Parker BD, Frederick RW, Reilly TP, Lowry PS, Bird ET. Efficiency and cost of treating proximal ureteral stones: shock wave lithotripsy versus ureteroscopy plus holmium:yttrium-aluminum-garnet laser. Urology. 2004;64(6):1102–6.
76. Wu CF, Shee JJ, Lin WY, Lin CL, Chen CS. Comparison between extracorporeal shock wave lithotripsy and semirigid ureterorenoscope with holmium: YAG laser lithotripsy for treating large proximal ureteral stones. J Urol. 2004;172(5 Pt 1):1899–902.
77. Verze P, Imbimbo C, Cancelmo G, Creta M, Palmieri A, Mangiapia F, Buonopane R, Mirone V. Extracorporeal shockwave lithotripsy vs ureteroscopy as first-line therapy for patients with single distal ureteric stones: a prospective randomized study. BJU Int. 2010;106(11): 1745–52.
78. Hendrikx AJ, Strijbos WE, de Knijff DW, Kums JJ, Doesburg WH, Lemmens WA. Treatment for extended-mid and distal ureteral stones: SWL or ureteroscopy? Results of a multicenter study. J Endourol. 1999;13(10):727–33.
79. Peschel R, Janetschek G, Bartsch G. Extracorporeal shock wave lithotripsy versus ureteroscopy for distal ureteral calculi: a prospective randomized study. J Urol. 1999;162(6): 1909–12.
80. Egilmez T, Tekin MI, Gonen M, Kilinc F, Goren R, Ozkardes H. Efficacy and safety of a new-generation shockwave lithotripsy machine in the treatment of single renal or ureteral stones: experience with 2,670 patients. J Endourol. 2007;21(1):23–7.
81. De Sio M, Autorino R, Quarto G, Mordente S, Giugliano F, di Giacomo F, Neri F, Quattrone C, Sorrentino D, De Domenico R, D'Armientro M. A new transportable shock-wave lithotripsy machine for managing urinary stones: a single-centre experience with a dual-focus lithotripter. BJU Int. 2007;100(5):1137–41.
82. Murota-Kawano A, Ohya K, Sekine H. Outpatient basis extracorporeal shock wave lithotripsy for ureter stones: efficacy of the third generation lithotripter as the first line treatment. Int J Urol. 2008;15(3):210–5.
83. Tiselius HG. How efficient is extracorporeal shockwave lithotripsy with modern lithotripters for removal of ureteral stones? J Endourol. 2008;22(2):249–55.
84. Seitz C, Martini T, Berner L, Signorello D, Galantini A, Pycha A. Efficacy and treatment outcome of a new electromagnetic lithotripter for upper urinary tract calculi. J Endourol. 2008;22(11):2519–25.

Chapter 5
Observation and Medical Expulsive Therapy

Sara L. Best

Introduction

The prevalence of nephrolithiasis has been estimated at 1–15 %, with 10–15 % of Americans receiving this diagnosis over the course of a lifetime [1]. In 2000, it was estimated that over $2 billion was spent on the treatment of urolithiasis, a 46 % increase from 1994 expenditures [2]. Much of the morbidity of kidney stone disease pertains to the risks associated with ureterolithiasis, including renal colic and the potential for long-term renal damage from obstruction. Prior to the advent of safe and effective minimally-invasive surgical therapies for ureteral stones, the only alternative to spontaneous stone passage was frequently open ureterolithotomy. With the rise of endourology and techniques such as shockwave lithotripsy, ureteroscopy, and percutaneous nephrostolithotomy, the morbidity of stone surgery has dramatically decreased, but there remains a role for a non-surgical approach in many cases. Miller and Kane, for example, found that 83 % of stones passed spontaneously without intervention [3]. While stone passage rates can be favorable, there remains room for improvement to avoid surgical morbidity and cost, leaving a role for medical expulsive therapy (MET). Additionally, though a stone may ultimately pass, there can be prolonged morbidity such as pain, risk of infection, and lifestyle disruption during the passage interval. Thus therapy to improve time to stone passage is also desirable. The following chapter will review the physiology of ureteral obstruction as well as the observational and medical expulsive therapeutic agents and literature.

S.L. Best, MD
Department of Urology, University of Wisconsin School of Medicine and Public Health, Madison, WI, USA
e-mail: best@urology.wisc.edu

S.R. Patel, S.Y. Nakada (eds.), *Ureteral Stone Management: A Practical Approach*, DOI 10.1007/978-3-319-08792-4_5

Observation

Observation without surgical intervention is often a reasonable initial approach to ureterolithiasis, as most small ureteral stones will pass spontaneously without surgical intervention. A meta-analysis conducted by the American Urological Association/ European Association of Urology Nephrolithiasis Guideline Panel estimated that the median probability of stone passage was 68 % for stones ≤5 mm (n=224) and 47 % for those >5 and ≤10 mm (n=104) in size [4]. Other studies have suggested even higher rates of passage, particularly for distal ureteral stones. Ibrahim and colleagues reported stone passage rates of 71–98 % for stones <5 mm in size [5]. The majority of stones pass spontaneously within 4–6 weeks. This was demonstrated by Miller and Kane, who reported that of stones ≤2 mm, 2–4 mm and 4–6 mm in size, 95 % of those which passed did so by 31, 40, and 39 days, respectively [3]. Notably, the majority of the stones in this study were found in the distal ureter.

One of the feared complications of conservative management of ureteric stones is the "silent loss" of renal function. Andren-Sandberg prospectively monitored renal function with radioisotope renography in 358 consecutive patients with ureteral stones until each patient was stone-free [6]. He reported impaired renal function at presentation in 91 patients. In 24 of these patients – 7 % of the total series – the impairment was still present after the latest examination, on average 17 months after stone clearance, though the author noted the degree of impairment to be mild in most cases (numerical data not provided). The study found that the patients most at risk for persistent loss of renal function were patients with large stones, long duration of stone presence in the ureter, elderly patients and women.

Kelleher and coauthors also studied the impact of ureteral calculi on renal function by obtaining ^{99m}Tc-DTPA renography in 76 patients with ureteral stones <10 mm [7]. All patients were found to be obstructed at the time of admission on intravenous urography (IVU). They obtained nuclear scans within 24 h of admission then every 72–96 h until the stone had passed or the obstruction surgically relieved. Follow up scans were obtained 3 months after discharge and no patient was left obstructed >7 days. Interestingly, only 51 % of patients were still obstructed on the renographic study obtained within 24 h of the IVU, highlighting the dynamic (and potentially unpredictable) nature of obstruction from ureteral stones. The authors found that renal split function returned to normal after stone removal in all patients but two, both of whom had function <25 % upon presentation and had been treated for large stones in the past which may have caused the renal damage.

Roberts and colleagues retrospectively evaluated 21 patients with ureteral stones that had been impacted for 2–48 months (mean 8.8 months), described as a "series of 'worst-case' obstructions" [8]. Follow-up IVU or isotope renography revealed ureteral strictures in five patients (24 %), all of whom had had at least 5 months of impaction (mean 11 months). Additionally, four-fifths of these patients had a history of iatrogenic ureteral perforation from failed prior intervention. In the other 16 patients, intravenous urography or nuclear-medicine studies were normal after stone removal.

Hubner et al. found the risk of complications including ureteral stricture, sepsis, and increased technical difficulty during subsequent surgical treatment reached 20 % when symptoms exceeded 4 weeks in duration, compared to 7 % [9].

Most authors recommend that a trial of stone passage, with or without MET, should be limited to 4–6 weeks even in the patient with well-controlled symptoms due to the risk of renal damage or other complications [10, 11]. Additionally, tolerance of complications from unpassed stones has understandably diminished as surgical therapies for ureteral calculi have become more successful and less morbid.

The Physiology of Ureteral Contractility

Prior to delving into the potential targets for medical expulsive therapy, it is helpful to understand the normal conduction of urine from kidney to bladder and the physiologic response to obstruction, such as from a ureteral calculus. The collecting system and ureter contain syncytial-type smooth muscle, which depend on cell-to-cell transmission of excitation via neurotransmitters rather than neuromuscular junctions. The smooth muscle cells depolarize, calcium flows into the cells and contraction occurs. Thus, upper tract peristalsis can occur in the absence of innervation. Contractions in the calices and renal pelvis are more frequent and stronger than those in the ureter and this is thought to promote the antegrade flow of urine [12]. Pacemaker cells in the renal pelvis are thought to regulate this process.

While upper tract contractility is not dependent on innervation, both the parasympathetic and sympathetic autonomic nervous systems influence ureteral activity [13]. Alpha receptor stimulation triggers ureteral contraction while beta receptor stimulation promotes relaxation.

The physiologic response to unilateral ureteral obstruction is time dependent. In the first 1–2 h, renal blood flow increases and there is a build-up of urine that cannot bypass the obstruction, resulting in increased pressure within the collecting system. This pressure eventually declines around 5 h after obstruction as renal blood flow declines [14]. In response to the high pressure, the ureteral wall expends its force to maintenance of wall tone and cannot generate peristalsis, resulting in the loss of active transport of urine [15]. Both ureteral length and diameter increase in proximal to the site of obstruction [16].

The main physiologic reactions thought to slow or prevent ureteral stone passage include ureteral spasm and edema induced by the presence of a calculus. These reactions present potential targets for pharmacotherapy. An ideal agent would reduce ureteral edema and spasm while preserving peristalsis, which is thought to promote stone migration. A number of pharmacologic agents with these potential actions have been studied in vitro or in animal models.

Page and colleagues conducted a randomized swine study to evaluate the effects of alpha blockade during ureteral obstruction [17]. Twenty-four animals were divided into four groups including a control group without α-blockade or ureteral obstruction, a group with alfuzosin α-blockade and no ureteral obstruction, a cohort without α-blockade but with distal ureteral obstruction, and a group with α-blockade and distal obstruction. Ureteral pressures were then measured. The authors reported a significant increase in ureteral pressure and peristaltic rate with distal ureteral obstruction. Overall, there was no effect seen in these parameters with medication, but they did note a trend towards a decrease in the peristaltic pressure change in the treated obstructed group of 0.2 mmHg (95 % confidence interval: −0.55 −0.10; $p=0.06$).

An in vitro investigation conducted by Nakada et al. found that exposure to doxazosin reduced spontaneous ureteral contractility in a dose-dependent fashion as well as increased relaxation when the ureter was exposed to epinephrine [18].

Ames and coauthors also measured porcine ureteral peristalsis in an in vivo experiment exposing the ureter to topical theophylline or verapamil [19]. They found that theophylline inhibited ureteral peristalsis and verapamil produced acute proximal-ureteral dilation of 1.17 mm more than the control ($p=0.03$).

Studies such as these indicate the complexity of ureteral physiology, suggesting a potential role for drugs across a wide variety of pharmacologic classes as medical expulsive therapy.

Agents Used as Medical Expulsive Therapy

Alpha Blockers

Medications that block α-1 adrenergic receptor activity, commonly referred to as "alpha blockers," are the most-studied medical expulsive agents. This class of drugs, commonly used in the management of symptomatic benign prostatic hyperplasia, is thought to improve stone passage rates by inhibiting the α-1 adrenergic receptor-mediated ureteral spasm induced by calculi. A number of agents within this class, both selective and non-selective, have been investigated as MET, including doxazosin, terazosin, tamsulosin, alfuzosin, and silodosin. Studies suggest efficacy of all of these medications in promoting stone passage. While doxazosin and terazosin are less expensive than the other alpha blockers, the receptor selectivity of the other three agents may lead to fewer side effects, such as hypotension or lightheadedness (Table 5.1). Another important side effect of this class is *Intraoperative Floppy Iris Syndrome*, which has been observed during cataract surgery even months after discontinuing drug therapy [20]. This syndrome is associated with a higher risk of cataract surgical complications, though modifications of surgical technique can be helpful if planned for. Initiation of alpha blocker therapy should therefore be avoided in patients with upcoming cataract surgery.

In 2002, Cervenakov and colleagues published the first study of alpha antagonists as medical expulsive therapy to appear in the literature [21]. In this double-blinded study, the investigators randomized 104 patients with distal ureteral stones to standard therapy or standard therapy plus tamsulosin 0.4 mg daily. While no statistical analysis was done, the authors reported improved stone passage rates in the group receiving tamsulosin (80 % vs. 63 %), as well as faster stone passage. These findings prompted further investigations into these agents.

Table 5.1 Medical expulsive therapy potential side effects

Agent class	Drugs in class reported in MET studies	Proposed mechanism of action	Safety in pregnancy	Potential side effects[a]
Selective COX inhibitors	Celecoxib	Inhibition of COX-2 enzymes, reduction of ureteral contractility	Class C (risk cannot be ruled out) [a]may cause premature closure of the fetal patent ductus arteriosus	GI: upset, ulcers/bleeding
				Renal: ↓renal blood flow, renal insufficiency
				CV: ↑risk of MI and stroke, hypertension
NSAIDs/ Non-selective COX inhibitors	Indomethacin, ibuprofen, diclofenac	Inhibition of COX-1 and 2 enzymes, reduction of ureteral contractility	Class C (risk cannot be ruled out) [a]may cause premature closure of the fetal patent ductus arteriosus	GI: upset, ulcers/bleeding
				Renal: ↓ renal blood flow, renal insufficiency
				CV: ↑risk of MI and stroke, hypertension
Steroids	Methylprednisolone, deflazacort, prednisone	Anti-inflammatory, reduction of ureteral edema	Class C (risk cannot be ruled out)	CV: arrhythmias, thromboembolism
				CNS: emotional disturbance
				Endocrine: adrenal suppression, hyperglycemia
				GI: hemorrhage, ulcer, ↑transaminases
				Misc: leukocytosis, osteoporosis, impaired wound healing, cataracts, aseptic joint necrosis, infections
Calcium-channel blockers	Nifedipine	Calcium channel blockade impairs depolarization of smooth muscle cells in ureter, promoting relaxation	Class C (risk cannot be ruled out)	CV: flushing, edema, palpitations, hypotension
				CNS: dizziness, headache, fatigue
				GI: nausea

(continued)

Table 5.1 (continued)

Agent class	Drugs in class reported in MET studies	Proposed mechanism of action	Safety in pregnancy	Potential side effects[a]
Alpha-blockers	Tamsulosin, doxazosin, terazosin, silodosin	Alpha adrenergic receptor blockade, ureteral smooth muscle relaxation, ↓ureteral peristalsis	Tamsulosin, alfuzosin and silodosin: Class B (adverse events not observed in animal reproduction studies) [a]these drugs are not FDA-labeled for use in women	CV: orthostatic hypotension
			Doxazosin and terazosin: Class C (risk cannot be ruled out)	CNS: headache, dizziness, fatigue
				ENT: rhinitis, Intraoperative Floppy Iris Syndrome
				GU: Abnormal ejaculation
Anticholinergics	Tolteridine, oxybutynin	Smooth muscle relaxation via muscarinic receptors	Oxybutynin: Class B (adverse events not observed in animal reproduction studies)	CV: hypertension
			Tolteridine: Class C (risk cannot be ruled out)	CNS: cognitive changes, especially in elderly
				ENT: dry mucous membranes, glaucoma
				GI: constipation
				GU: urinary retention

CV cardiovascular, *CNS* central nervous system, *ENT* ear, nose, and throat, *GI* gastrointestinal, *GU* genitourinary

[a]List of side effects is not meant to be fully inclusive and medication inserts and other sources should be consulted for a full listing before prescribing these drugs

Since that time, dozens of studies on the effect of alpha blockers on stone passage have appeared in the literature, too many to individually review here. The abundance of investigations has allowed several meta-analyses to be conducted, summarizing the findings of these studies. The outcomes of these meta-analyses can be found in Table 5.2. The first meta-analysis published was by Hollingsworth and colleagues in 2006 [22]. When the authors excluded studies in which patients also received either steroids or benzodiazepines, they calculated that alpha blockers were associated with a 54 % increase in stone passage compared to control (RR 1.54; $P<0.001$; 95 % CI 1.29–1.85).

The combined American Urological Association/European Association of Urology Nephrolithiasis Guideline Panel included a discussion of the role of MET in their 2007 Guideline for the Management of Ureteral Calculi [4]. In this document, the panelists summarized a meta-analysis of the six alpha blocker RCTs available at that time by stating that alpha antagonists were associated with a 29 % absolute increase in stone passage rates compared to control, which was statistically significant.

Beyond improving stone passage rates, alpha blockers may also decrease pain associated with ureterolithiasis. Sayed and colleagues randomized 90 patients with distal ureteral stones to either analgesia on-demand with diclofenac or tamsulosin + analgesia [23]. In addition to an absolute increase in stone passage of 38 %, tamsulosin use was associated with a decrease in number of renal colic episodes (1.5 vs 2.5 episodes, $p=0.003$) and a decreased use of analgesics (0.14 vs 2.7 vials, $p<0.0001$). Porpiglia et al. investigated the role of both tamsulosin and corticosteroids in a 2006 study where they randomized 114 patients to tamsulosin, deflazacort 30 mg daily, both, or analgesia only [24]. While both groups taking tamsulosin experienced significantly higher rates of stone passage, only the group receiving combination therapy with tamsulosin and deflazacort consumed significantly less analgesic than the control group (27 mg vs 81 mg diclofenac, $p<0.001$).

Finally, medical expulsive therapy with alpha antagonists may speed stone passage. De Sio and coauthors randomized 96 patients with distal ureteral stones (mean 6.4–6.9 mm) to either diclofenac + aescin (control group) or control therapy + tamsulosin [25] They found the stone passage rate at 2 weeks to be significantly higher in the tamsulosin group (90 % vs. 59 %, $p=0.01$) but also noted the alpha blocker was associated with faster stone passage (mean 4.4 vs. 7.5 days, $p=0.005$). Other studies have since reported similar findings, summarized by Lu et al. where meta-analysis of 16 studies showed a shorter mean expulsion time with alpha blockers by 3.4 days (95 % CI −4.5 to −2.29 days) [26].

Calcium Channel Blockers

Calcium channel blockers (CCBs) are the most studied medical expulsive agents after alpha blockers. CCBs have been shown to inhibit ureteral contraction and may inhibit spasm without affecting ureteral peristalsis [27, 28]. Drugs in this class that

Table 5.2 Published meta-analyses of alpha-blocker agents for medical expulsive therapy

Study/year published	# Studies included	# Patients included	Alpha-blockers included	Effect on stone passage rates	Effect on time to stone passage	Additional findings
Hollingsworth 2006 [22]	5	[a]	Tamsulosin, doxazosin, terazosin (steroids and benzodiazepines excluded)	Alpha blockers improved rates of stone passage (RR 1.54; $P<0.001$; 95 % CI 1.29–1.85)	NR (data not pooled)	
Preminger 2007 [4]	6	280	Tamsulosin, doxazosin, terazosin (potentially confounding agents in included studies: steroids)	29 % absolute increase in stone passage rates with alpha blockers	NR	
Singh 2007 [50]	16	1,235	Tamsulosin (13/16), doxazosin, terazosin (potentially confounding agents in included studies: steroids, anticholinergics)	Alpha-blockers improved rates of stone passage (RR 1.59; 95 % CI 1.44–1.75)	NR	Adverse events reported in 4 % of participants
Seitz 2009 [51]	29	2,419	Tamsulosin, doxazosin, terazosin, alfuzosin (potentially confounding agents in included studies: steroids, anticholinergics)	Alpha-blockers improved rates of stone passage: RR 1.45; 95 % CI 1.34–1.57 After excluding studies with potentially confounding drugs other than NSAIDs: RR 1.45; 95 % CI 1.31–1.45	NR (data not pooled)	Noted that few studies reported on adverse events

Lu 2012 [26]	29	2,763	Tamsulosin (potentially confounding agents in included studies: steroids, anticholinergics benzodiazepines)	19 % improved stone passage rate with tamsulosin	Shorter mean expulsion time by 3.4 days than control group (based on 16 studies) (95 % CI –4.5 to –2.29 days)	Reduced colic (based on eight studies): WMD=0–0.44 episodes, 95 % CI –0.76 to –0.12)
Fan 2013 [52]	20	1,593	Tamsulosin	Lower ureteral stones: P<0.00001; RR 1.55; 95 % CI 1.43–1.68	Shorter mean expulsion time by 2.63 days than control group (based on 7 studies): P<00001,95 % CI –4.13 to –3.12 days)	Reduced colic (based on five studies): P=0.0003, RR 0.60, 95 % CI 0.45–0.79)
	Did not separate studies using MET as adjunct to SWL			Upper ureteral stones: P=0.02; RR 1.28; 95 % CI: 1.04–1.57		Alpha blockers associated with higher risk of side effects (based on eight studies, P=0.0007; RR 2.17; 95 % CI 1.39–3.40) (most common = dizziness)
				All locations: P<0.0001; RR 1.51; 95 % CI 1.40–1.63		

RR relative risk, *CI* confidence interval, *NR* not reported, *WMD* weighted mean distribution

[a]Exact number of patients for alpha blocker studies not reported

have been studied as MET include nifedipine, diltiazem, and verapamil, though clinical trials have almost exclusively employed nifedipine.

Most of the early studies of nifedipine as MET included combination therapy with an oral steroid agent. For example Borghi and colleagues' study randomized 86 patients to receive either nifedipine and methylprednisolone or methylprednisolone alone and found a significantly faster and higher stone passage rates in the nifedipine/steroid combination group than steroid alone (87 % vs. 65 %, $p=0.021$) [29]. Cooper and colleagues reported similar findings comparing nifedipine and prednisone to analgesia alone (stone passage rates of 86 % vs 54 %, $p=0.001$) [30]. The results of similar studies can be found in Table 5.3.

While most of these early studies suggest efficacy of a CCB/steroid combination, more recent studies comparing CCB monotherapy and alpha blockers head-to-head have found alpha blockers to be the superior agents. Dellabella and colleagues randomized patients to phloroglucinol (a steroid), tamsulosin, or nifedipine and found tamsulosin to be the most efficacious agent to promote stone passage (97 % vs. 64 % and 77 %, $p=0.001$ and <0.0001), despite the tamsulosin group having a statistically larger stone size [31]. Ye and coauthors had very similar findings in their study of 3,189 patients, comparing tamsulosin and nifedipine (96 % passage vs. 74 %, $p<0.01$) [32]. The meta-analysis conducted for the AUA Ureteral Stone Guideline included four studies and reported that nifedipine was associated with an absolute increase in stone passage rates of 8 %, which was not statistically significant.[4]

Additional Drugs Used for MET

Non-steroidal Anti-inflammatory Drugs (NSAIDs)

The prostanoids (prostaglandins and thromboxanes) appear to influence ureteral contractility. These mediators are produced by cyclooxygenase (COX) enzymes and COX-2, the inducible form, has been found to be induced by mucosal injury and stretching of the urinary tract [33].

NSAIDs, already frequently prescribed for analgesia in cases of renal colic, are an attractive class of medications to study for MET, due to their inhibition of COX enzymes. Indeed in vitro, these compounds have been demonstrated to inhibit ureteral contractility [34, 35].

However limited placebo-controlled studies of NSAIDs have not shown these agents to increase stone passage rates. Studies of non-selective NSAIDs by Kapoor et al. [36] (indomethacin) and Laerum et al. [37] (diclofenac) reported decreased narcotic use and pain compared to placebo but no improvement in stone passage rates or time to stone passage. Phillips and coauthors conducted a placebo-controlled double-blind RCT utilizing celecoxib in 53 patients with ureteral calculi <10 mm and similarly found no significant different in passage rates or time [38]. This investigation, however, reported no significant different in either pain scores or narcotic use amongst participants.

Table 5.3 Published randomized controlled trials of non-alpha blocker medical expulsive agents

Stud year published	Study size	Characteristics of stones	Study arms	Effect on stone passage rates	Effect on time to stone passage	Additional findings
Kapoor 1989 [36]	26	Ureteral stone (mean 3 mm)	1. Indomethacin suppository 50 mg 3×/day × 5 days max 2. Placebo	No significant difference in stone passage rates	No significant difference in time to stone passage	Indomethacin group had fewer colic episodes, fewer admissions for pain, and significantly lower narcotic use ($p<0.005$)
Borghi 1994 [29]	86	Ureteral stone ≤15 mm (mean 6.7 mm)	1. Methylprednisolone 16 mg/day 2. Methylprednisolone 16 mg/day + nifedipine 40 mg/day	Methylprednisolone + nifedipine group had higher stone passage rate (87 % vs. 65 %, $p=0.021$)	Faster time to expulsion in Methylprednisolone + nifedipine group (11 vs 16 days, $p=0.036$)	
Cooper 2000 [30]	70	Ureteral stone 2–6 mm (mean 3.9 mm)	1. Nifedipine XL 30 mg/day (max 7 days) + prednisone 20 mg/day (max 5 days) + trimethoprim sulfa 2. Analgesia	Treatment group associated with a higher stone passage rate than analgesia alone (86 % vs 54 %, $p=0.001$)	No difference in time to stone passage	Fewer lost days of work in treatment group (1.8 vs 5.0, p-0.024)
Porpiglia 2000 [53]	96	Single distal stone ≤10 mm (mean 5.5–5.8 mm)	1. Deflazacort 30 mg/day (max 10 day) and nifedipine 30 mg/day (max 28 days) 2. Analgesia alone	Deflazacort/nifedipine group had higher stone passage rate (79 % vs. 35 %, $p<0.05$)	Faster time to expulsion in treatment group (7 vs 20 days, $p<0.05$)	Lower consumption of analgesics in treatment group (15 vs. 105 mg of diclofenac, $p<0.05$)

(continued)

Table 5.3 (continued)

Stud year published	Study size	Characteristics of stones	Study arms	Effect on stone passage rates	Effect on time to stone passage	Additional findings
Porpiglia 2004 [54]	86	Single distal stone <10 mm (mean 4.7–5.4 mm)	1. Deflazacort 30 mg/day (max 10 day) and nifedipline 30 mg/day (max 28 days)	Both treatment groups had higher stone passage rate (80 % and 85 % vs 43 %, p<0.01)	Faster time to expulsion in deflazacort + tamsulosin group than analgesia alone (8 vs 12 days, p=0.02)	Lower consumption of analgesics in both treatment groups (20 and 26 vs. 105 mg of diclofenac, p<0.0001)
			2. Deflazacort 30 mg/day (max 10 day) and tamsulosin 0.4 mg/day (max 28 days)			
			3. Analgesia alone			
Saita 2004 [40]	50	Ureteral stone ≤15 mm (mean 12 mm)	1. Nifedipine slow release 30 mg/day (max 20 day.) and Prednisolone 25 mg/day (max 10 day)	Stone passage 68 % in nifedipine group, 81 % in prednisolone group	NR	
			2. Prednisolone 25 mg/day (max 10 day)			
Dellabella 2005 [31]	210	Single distal stone ≥4 mm (mean 6.2–7.2 mm)	1. Phloroglucinol 240 mg/day	Tamsulosin associated with higher stone passage rates (97 % vs. 64 % and 77 %, p=0.001 and <0.0001)	Faster time to expulsion in tamsulosin group (72 vs. 120 and 120 h, p=0.001 and <0.0001)	Better pain control and fewer hospitalizations in tamsulosin group
		Tamsulosin group had statistically larger stones	2. Tamsulosin 0.4 mg/day	No difference between phloroglucinol and nifedipine (p=0.19)	No difference between phloroglucinol and nifedipine (p=0.455)	
			3. Nifedipine slow release 30 mg/day			

Erturhan 2007 [41]	120	Ureteral stone <10 mm (mean 7 mm)	1. Tamsulosin 0.4 mg/day 2. Tamsulosin 0.4 mg/day + tolterodine 2 mg 2×/day 3. Tolterodine 2 mg 2×/day 4. Analgesia alone	Both tamsulosin groups had higher stone passage rate than tolterodine or analgesia alone (73 % and 70 % vs 47 % and 40 %, $p<0.05$)	Faster time to explusion in both tamsulosin groups than tolterodine or analgesia alone (6 and 8 vs 11 and 12 days, $p<0.05$)	Pain and analgesic use significantly less in both tamsulosin groups
Preminger 2007 [4]	160	Meta-analysis of four studies	Meta-analysis of four studies using nifedipine	Nifedipine associated with an absolute increase in stone passage rates of 8 % (not statistically significant)	NR	
Phillips 2009 [38]	53	Obstructing ureteral calculus <10 mm (mean 4.8 mm)	1. Celecoxib 400 mg × 1, then 200 mg 2×/day × 10 day 2. Placebo	No significant difference in stone passage rates (55 % vs 54 %, $p=0.69$)	No significant difference in time to stone passage (7 vs. 9 days, $p=0.6$)	No significant difference in pain scores or narcotic doses
Ye 2011 [32]	3,189	Single distal stone (mean 5.7 mm)	1. Tamsulosin 0.4 mg/day 2. Nifedipine 10 mg/3 times/day	Tamsulosin associated with higher stone passage rates (96 % vs. 74 %, $p<0.01$)	Faster time to expulsion in tamsulosin group (78 vs. 138 h, $p<0.01$)	Lower consumption of analgesics in tamsulosin group (52 vs. 109 mg of diclofenac, $p<0.01$)
Lv 2013 [42]	103	Intramural ureteral stone 4–9 mm (mean 7 mm) and "vesical irritability"	1. Tamsulosin 0.4 mg/day 2. Tamsulosin 0.4 mg/day + tolterodine 2 mg 2×/day 3. Tolterodine 2 mg 2×/day	Both groups taking tamsulosin had higher stone passage rate than tolterodine alone (81 % and 85 % vs 56 %, $p=0.003$)	Faster time to explusion in both tamsulosin groups than tolterodine alone (8 vs 11 days, $p=0.000$)	Both tolterodine groups reported lower pain and urinary sensation scores and fewer pain episodes ($p<0.05$)

Steroids

The anti-inflammatory action of corticosteroids has made them appealing agents to use as medical expulsive therapy. Reducing ureteral edema and inflammation could promote stone passage. Hydrocortisone has also been shown to inhibit ureteral contractility in vitro [39].

Despite these theoretical advantages, the efficacy of steroids in promoting ureteral stone passage has been unclear. Few studies have randomized patients to steroid monotherapy and instead most have prescribed corticosteroids in conjunction with another expulsive agent such as a calcium channel blocker or alpha blocker, making the impact of the steroid unclear.

Borghi and colleagues randomized 86 patients to receive either methylprednisolone alone or in combination with nifedipine and found that combination therapy was associated with higher stone passage rates (87 % vs. 65 %, $p=0.021$) [29]. There was no placebo group, however, so the independent effect of the corticosteroid could not be assessed.

An investigation by Porpiglia et al. randomized 114 patients with distal ureteral stones (mean 5.8 mm) to the alpha blocker tamsulosin, deflazacort (a steroid), or combination therapy for 10 days and compared them to a control group receiving only analgesia [24]. Combination therapy proved more effective at improving stone passage at 10 days than either tamsulosin or deflazacort alone or placebo (85 % vs. 60 %, 38 %, and 33 %, respectively, $p<0.001$). Analgesic consumption was also lowest in the combination group ($p<0.001$).

Saita and coauthors enrolled 50 patients with larger ureteral stones (mean 12 mm) in a randomized controlled trial comparing 10 days of prednisolone (25 mg) plus up to 20 days therapy with nifedipine (30 mg) to prednisolone alone [40]. Despite the large average stone size, the authors reported stone passage rates of 81 and 68 %, respectively (p value not reported).

Despite these studies suggesting steroids may provide a synergistic effect with other forms of MET, many of the most recent publications do not include steroid therapy. This may be in part due to urologists' relative unfamiliarity with using steroid medications and concerns about side effects and dosing.

Anticholinergic Medications

The success of alpha-blockers as medical expulsive therapy has sparked an interest in other agents known to relax smooth muscle within the urinary tract. Anticholinergic medications may be particularly appealing to urologists, given their familiarity and comfort with using these drugs for overactive bladder.

Erturhan and colleagues hypothesized that anticholinergics could promote the passage of distal ureteral stones by relaxing the detrusor muscle, particularly the intramural tunnel [41]. To this end, they randomized 120 patients with distal stones to one of four groups: tamsulosin monotherapy, tolterodine monotherapy, combination therapy with tamsulosin and tolterodine, or placebo. Both groups taking tamsulosin experienced significantly higher and faster rates of stone passage as well as fewer bouts of renal colic than the tolterodine or placebo groups (73 % and 70 % stone passage rate vs 47 % and 40 %). Thus, they concluded that tolterodine provided no medical expulsive benefit.

Lv and Tang also randomized patients with intramural ureteral stones to receive tolterodine, tamsulosin, or dual therapy and similarly found that tolterodine alone group experienced a lower and slower stone passage rate than the two tamsulosin-containing groups [42]. However the tolterodine groups experienced significantly less urinary urgency, which can be a symptom associated with intramural stones.

While studies assessing anticholinergic medications as MET are few and, to date, only utilized tolterodine, the role for these drugs in promoting stone passage appears limited except as an adjunct in patients with vesical irritability.

MET and the Pediatric Population

While the only FDA-labeled indication for tamsulosin remains benign prostatic hyperplasia in men, there is precedent in the literature for using alpha-adrenergic antagonists in the pediatric urologic population in certain neurogenic bladder and voiding dysfunction patients [43]. Despite the success of shockwave lithotripsy and the miniaturization of endoscopes that now permits instrumentation of the pediatric upper tracts, avoidance of surgery remains desirable in the pediatric population and has prompted investigations into using MET in children.

Tasian and coauthors performed a retrospective case match study evaluating the outcomes children with ureteral stones prescribed either tamsulosin or analgesics alone [44]. Ninety-nine patients who had received tamsulosin were case matched with 99 children receiving analgesia alone. The mean age in this study was older, 14 years and mean stone size was 4 mm. They reported that 55 % of the cohort taking tamsulosin passed their stones compared to 44 % in the analgesia alone cohort ($p=0.03$) and no adverse side effects were noted.

Mokhless and colleagues randomized 61 children (mean age 8.1 years) with distal ureteral stones to receive either tamsulosin or placebo [45]. Dosing of tamsulosin was 0.4 mg nightly for children older than 4 years and 0.2 mg for younger children. Similar to studies in adults, tamsulosin was associated with statistically significant improvements in stone passage rates (88 % vs 64 %, $p<0.01$), time to passage (8 days vs 14.5, $p<0.001$), and pain. They also noted that no patient stopped the therapy due to side effects and they concluded tamsulosin was safe and effective as MET in children.

Who Should Get MET and How Is MET Used

MET is typically not the best initial treatment choice in patients with a solitary kidney, significant acute kidney injury, persistent pain or symptoms, or urinary tract infection. Also, due to the low chance of stone passage, MET may not be the best single treatment option in patients with large ureteral stones. However MET could be considered for use in the interval prior to planned elective surgical intervention in patients with well-controlled symptoms despite the low passage rate, given its additional impact on pain (discussed earlier).

Cost of MET

Issues of cost are complicated to analyze due to considerations of perspective (Cost to whom? The patient? The payer? Society?) as well as direct and indirect costs, which are not always easy to measure [46]. Despite these challenges, a brief discussion of cost is merited and timely, given recent political and societal focus on the rising costs of health care. Due to the high cost of surgery in the United States, it is easy to envision how successful stone passage with medical expulsive therapy could be associated with significant cost savings. In their decision tree model analysis, Bensalah, Pearle and Lotan reported that MET was associated with a $1,132 cost savings over observation in the United States [47]. Indeed, due to the low cost of medication (calculated at $28 in their model) compared to ureteroscopy ($4,973), MET was associated with cost savings even if the medication only improved stone passage rates by 1 %.

Dauw and colleagues determined that MET is also associated with *indirect* cost savings compared to early endoscopic stone surgery [48]. In their matched cohort analysis, the patients treated with medical expulsive therapy had a 6 % predicted probability of filing a claim for short-term disability compared to 16.5 % in the early endoscopic stone removal cohort ($p<0.0001$).

Brede and colleagues found that patients seen in the emergency room with renal colic who were treated with MET had a lower frequency of adverse outcomes (defined as repeat visits, hospitalization, or surgery, 37.7 % vs 53.1 %) and a lower mean total cost per patient ($1,805 vs $2,372) [49]. The authors used this information to help support an initiative to increase education of emergency department staff on the use of MET.

Future Directions

While existing literature shows promise regarding the role of medical expulsive therapy, future research may help elucidate which patients may benefit most from treatment, as well as determine which drug or combination of drugs is the most effective. Other recommendations such as how long of a course of MET to prescribe may be further defined. And finally, ongoing research is also taking place to determine to role of medical expulsive therapy as an adjunct to surgical therapy such as ureteroscopy and shockwave lithotripsy.

Take Home Points

- Many ureteral stones may pass and thus there is often a role for a carefully-monitored trial of observation, with or without medical expulsive therapy
- Ureteral physiology and the response to obstruction is complex, paving the way for a variety of medications to potentially manipulate stone passage
- Alpha blockers appear to be the most-efficacious single agents for MET
- MET may provide additional benefits beyond increased stone passage rates, such as reduced pain episodes

References

1. Pearle MS, Lotan Y, Wein AJ, Kovoussi LR, Novick AC, Partin AW, Peters CA. Campbell-Walsh urolog. In: Urinary Lithiasis. 10th ed. Philadelphia: Elsevier Saunders; 2012. Chapter 45.
2. Pearle MS, Calhoun E, Curhan G. Urolithiasis. In: Litwin M, Saigal C, US Department of Health and Human Services, Public Health Service, National Institutes of Health, National Institute of Diabetes and Digestive and Kidney Diseases, editors. Urologic diseases in America. Washington, DC: US Government Printing Office; 2007. p. 282–319.
3. Miller OF, Kane CJ. Time to stone passage for observed ureteral calculi: a guide for patient education. J Urol. 1999;162(3 Pt 1):688–90. discussion 90–1.
4. Preminger GM, Tiselius H-G, Assimos DG, et al. 2007 Guideline for the management of ureteral calculi. J Urol. 2007;178:2418–34.
5. Ibrahim AI, Shetty SD, Awad RM, Patel KP. Prognostic factors in the conservative treatment of ureteric stones. Br J Urol. 1991;67(4):358–61.
6. Andren-Sandberg A. Permanent impairment of renal function demonstrated by renographic follow-up in ureterolithiasis. Scand J Urol Nephrol. 1983;17(1):81–4.
7. Kelleher JP, Plail RO, Dave SM, Cunningham DA, Snell ME, Witherow RO. Sequential renography in acute urinary tract obstruction due to stone disease. Br J Urol. 1991;67(2):125–8.
8. Roberts WW, Cadeddu JA, Micali S, Kavoussi LR, Moore RG. Ureteral stricture formation after removal of impacted calculi. J Urol. 1998;159(3):723–6.
9. Hubner WA, Irby P, Stoller ML. Natural history and current concepts for the treatment of small ureteral calculi. Eur Urol. 1993;24(2):172–6.
10. Wang CJ, Huang SW, Chang CH. Medical expulsive therapy of ureteral stone. J Taiwan Urol Assoc. 2007;18(2):53–60.
11. Teichman JM. Clinical practice. Acute renal colic from ureteral calculus. N Engl J Med. 2004;350(7):684–93.
12. Morita T, Ishizuka G, Tsuchida S. Initiation and propagation of stimulus from the renal pelvic pacemaker in pig kidney. Invest Urol. 1981;19(3):157–60.
13. Santicioli P, Maggi CA. Myogenic and neurogenic factors in the control of pyeloureteral motility and ureteral peristalsis. Pharmacol Rev. 1998;50(4):683–722.
14. Moody TE, Vaughn Jr ED, Gillenwater JY. Relationship between renal blood flow and ureteral pressure during 18 hours of total unilateral uretheral occlusion. Implications for changing sites of increased renal resistance. Invest Urol. 1975;13(3):246–51.
15. Rose JG, Gillenwater JY. Effects of obstruction on ureteral function. Urology. 1978; 12(2):139–45.
16. Biancani P, Zabinski MP, Weiss RM. Bidimensional deformation of acutely obstructed in vitro rabbit ureter. Am J Physiol. 1973;225(3):671–4.

17. Page JB, Humphreys S, Davenport D, Crispen P, Venkatesh R. Second prize: in-vivo physiological impact of alpha blockade on the porcine ureter with distal ureteral obstruction. J Endourol. 2011;25(3):391–6.
18. Nakada SY, Coyle TL, Ankem MK, Moon TD, Jerde TJ. Doxazosin relaxes ureteral smooth muscle and inhibits epinephrine-induced ureteral contractility in vitro. Urology. 2007; 70(4):817–21.
19. Ames CD, Weld KJ, Dryer ST, Hruby G, Minor SD, Yan Y, et al. Pharmacologic manipulation of the porcine ureter: acute impact of topical drugs on ureteral diameter and peristaltic activity. J Endourol. 2006;20(11):943–8.
20. Abdel-Aziz S, Mamalis N. Intraoperative floppy iris syndrome. Curr Opin Ophthalmol. 2009;20(1):37–41.
21. Cervenakov I, Fillo J, Mardiak J, Kopecny M, Smirala J, Lepies P. Speedy elimination of ureterolithiasis in lower part of ureters with the alpha 1-blocker-tamsulosin. Int Urol Nephrol. 2002;34(1):25–9.
22. Hollingsworth JM, Rogers MA, Kaufman SR, Bradford TJ, Saint S, Wei JT, et al. Medical therapy to facilitate urinary stone passage: a meta-analysis. Lancet. 2006;368(9542):1171–9.
23. Sayed MA, Abolyosr A, Abdalla MA, El-Azab AS. Efficacy of tamsulosin in medical expulsive therapy for distal ureteral calculi. Scand J Urol Nephrol. 2008;42(1):59–62.
24. Porpiglia F, Vaccino D, Billia M, Renard J, Cracco C, Ghignone G, et al. Corticosteroids and tamsulosin in the medical expulsive therapy for symptomatic distal ureter stones: single drug or association. Eur Urol. 2006;50(2):339–44.
25. De Sio M, Autorino R, Di Lorenzo G, Damiano R, Giordano D, Cosentino L, et al. Medical expulsive treatment of distal-ureteral stones using tamsulosin: a single-center experience. J Endourol. 2006;20(1):12–6.
26. Lu Z, Dong Z, Ding H, Wang H, Ma B, Wang Z. Tamsulosin for ureteral stones: a systematic review and meta-analysis of a randomized controlled trial. Urol Int. 2012;89(1):107–15.
27. Hertle L, Nawrath H. Calcium channel blockade in smooth muscle of the human upper urinary tract. II. Effects on norepinephrine-induced activation. J Urol. 1984;132(6):1270–4.
28. Hertle L, Nawrath H. Calcium channel blockade in smooth muscle of the human upper urinary tract. I. Effects on depolarization-induced activation. J Urol. 1984;132(6):1265–9.
29. Borghi L, Meschi T, Amato F, Novarini A, Giannini A, Quarantelli C, et al. Nifedipine and methylprednisolone in facilitating ureteral stone passage: a randomized, double-blind, placebo-controlled study. J Urol. 1994;152(4):1095–8.
30. Cooper JT, Stack GM, Cooper TP. Intensive medical management of ureteral calculi. Urology. 2000;56(4):575–8.
31. Dellabella M, Milanese G, Muzzonigro G. Randomized trial of the efficacy of tamsulosin, nifedipine and phloroglucinol in medical expulsive therapy for distal ureteral calculi. J Urol. 2005;174(1):167–72.
32. Ye Z, Yang H, Li H, Zhang X, Deng Y, Zeng G, et al. A multicentre, prospective, randomized trial: comparative efficacy of tamsulosin and nifedipine in medical expulsive therapy for distal ureteric stones with renal colic. BJU Int. 2011;108(2):276–9.
33. Andersson KE, Arner A. Urinary bladder contraction and relaxation: physiology and pathophysiology. Physiol Rev. 2004;84(3):935–86.
34. Mastrangelo D, Wisard M, Rohner S, Leisinger H, Iselin CE. Diclofenac and NS-398, a selective cyclooxygenase-2 inhibitor, decrease agonist-induced contractions of the pig isolated ureter. Urol Res. 2000;28(6):376–82.
35. Jerde TJ, Calamon-Dixon JL, Bjorling DE, Nakada SY. Celecoxib inhibits ureteral contractility and prostanoid release. Urology. 2005;65(1):185–90.
36. Kapoor DA, Weitzel S, Mowad JJ, Melanson S, Gillen J. Use of indomethacin suppositories in the prophylaxis of recurrent ureteral colic. J Urol. 1989;142(6):1428–30.
37. Laerum E, Ommundsen OE, Gronseth JE, Christiansen A, Fagertun HE. Oral diclofenac in the prophylactic treatment of recurrent renal colic. A double-blind comparison with placebo. Eur Urol. 1995;28(2):108–11.

38. Phillips E, Hinck B, Pedro R, Makhlouf A, Kriedberg C, Hendlin K, et al. Celecoxib in the management of acute renal colic: a randomized controlled clinical trial. Urology. 2009; 74(5):994–9.
39. Bandi G, Wilkinson EA, Cary-Coyle TL, Jerde TJ, Nakada SY. Third prize: effect of hydrocortisone on porcine ureteral contractility in vitro. J Endourol. 2008;22(6):1169–73.
40. Saita A, Bonaccorsi A, Marchese F, Condorelli SV, Motta M. Our experience with nifedipine and prednisolone as expulsive therapy for ureteral stones. Urol Int. 2004;72 Suppl 1:43–5.
41. Erturhan S, Erbagci A, Yagci F, Celik M, Solakhan M, Sarica K. Comparative evaluation of efficacy of use of tamsulosin and/or tolterodine for medical treatment of distal ureteral stones. Urology. 2007;69(4):633–6.
42. Lv JL, Tang Q. Tamsulosin and tolterodine in the medical expulsive therapy for intramural ureteral stones with vesical irritability: a prospective randomized study. Urolithiasis. 2013; 41(5):417–21.
43. Husmann DA. Use of sympathetic alpha antagonists in the management of pediatric urologic disorders. Curr Opin Urol. 2006;16(4):277–82.
44. Tasian GE, Cost NG, Granberg CF, Pulido JE, Rivera M, Schwen Z, et al. Tamsulosin and spontaneous passage of ureteral stones in children: a multi-institutional cohort study. J Urol. 2014;192:506–1. Epub Feb 8, 2014.
45. Mokhless I, Zahran AR, Youssif M, Fahmy A. Tamsulosin for the management of distal ureteral stones in children: a prospective randomized study. J Pediatr Urol. 2012;8(5):544–8.
46. Lotan Y, Pearle MS. Economics of stone management. Urol Clin North Am. 2007; 34(3):443–53.
47. Bensalah K, Pearle M, Lotan Y. Cost-effectiveness of medical expulsive therapy using alpha-blockers for the treatment of distal ureteral stones. Eur Urol. 2008;53(2):411–8.
48. Dauw CA, Kaufman SR, Hollenbeck BK, Roberts WW, Faerber GJ, Wolf Jr JS, et al. Expulsive therapy versus early endoscopic stone removal in patients with acute renal colic: a comparison of indirect costs. J Urol. 2014;191(3):673–7.
49. Brede C, Hollingsworth JM, Faerber GJ, Taylor JS, Wolf Jr JS. Medical expulsive therapy for ureteral calculi in the real world: targeted education increases use and improves patient outcome. J Urol. 2010;183(2):585–9.
50. Singh A, Alter HJ, Littlepage A. A systematic review of medical therapy to facilitate passage of ureteral calculi. Ann Emerg Med. 2007;50(5):552–63.
51. Seitz C, Liatsikos E, Porpiglia F, Tiselius HG, Zwergel U. Medical therapy to facilitate the passage of stones: what is the evidence. Eur Urol. 2009;56(3):455–71.
52. Fan B, Yang D, Wang J, Che X, Li X, Wang L, et al. Can tamsulosin facilitate expulsion of ureteral stones? a meta-analysis of randomized controlled trials. Int J Urol. 2013;20(8): 818–30.
53. Porpiglia F, Destefanis P, Fiori C, Fontana D. Effectiveness of nifedipine and deflazacort in the management of distal ureter stones. Urology. 2000;56(4):579–82.
54. Porpiglia F, Ghignone G, Fiori C, Fontana D, Scarpa RM. Nifedipine versus tamsulosin for the management of lower ureteral stones. J Urol. 2004;172(2):568–71.

Chapter 6
Shock Wave Lithotripsy for the Treatment of Ureteral Stones

Marcel Hruza and Jens Rassweiler

Introduction

According to the American Urological Association (AUA)/European Association of Urology (EAU) "2007 guideline for the management of ureteral calculi", extracorporal shock wave lithotripsy (SWL) and ureteroscopy (URS) are the two primary treatment modalities to manage symptomatic ureteral stones when conservative treatment did not lead to spontaneous passage of the stone [1]. Open or laparoscopic stone surgery are secondary treatment options. Although open or laparoscopic stone surgery are only used in rare difficult cases in industrialized countries today, they remain an important alternative in emerging economies and developing countries [2]. The efficacy of extracorporeal shock wave lithotripsy for the treatment of ureteral calculi has been illustrated in the 1980s at the beginning of the SWL era [3]. In western countries, recent technological developments in endoscopy have caused an increase of endoscopic treatments for both renal and ureteral stones resulting in a decrease of SWL procedures [1]. Will there be a role for SWL in the future?

This chapter analyzes the potential utility and limitations of SWL for ureteral calculi, especially in comparison to endoscopic procedures. We will discuss which parameters have to be considered to achieve optimal outcomes of SWL, which complications lurk from SWL and how the risk of complications can be minimized.

M. Hruza, MD (✉) • J. Rassweiler, MD
Department of Urology, SLK Kliniken Heilbronn, University of Heidelberg, Am Gesundbrunnen 20-26, 74078 Heilbronn, Germany
e-mail: marcel.hruza@gmail.com; jens.rassweiler@slk-kliniken.de

S.R. Patel, S.Y. Nakada (eds.), *Ureteral Stone Management: A Practical Approach*, DOI 10.1007/978-3-319-08792-4_6

Performance of SWL for Ureteral Calculi

Contraindications of SWL

Contraindications of SWL for the treatment of ureteral as well as renal calculi include pregnancy, untreated urinary tract infections, untreated bleeding disorders as well as the use of oral anticoagulants, and large aortic aneurysms.

SWL in a patient with untreated bacteriuria may lead to a febrile urinary tract infection or even to urosepsis. Therefore, the urine of every patient should be screened for bacteriuria prior to SWL, for example with dipsticks. When bacteriuria is present, a urine culture and treatment with appropriate antibiotics is recommended. If the patient with bacteriuria has hydronephrosis due to an obstructing ureteral stone, we insert a double J stent or a percutaneous nephrostomy at the beginning of the antibiotic treatment to achieve good drainage of the infected urine from the kidney. This shortens the time to freedom from infection and minimizes the risk of urosepsis.

Patients taking oral anticoagulants without an adequate break before SWL treatment have an increased risk of hematuria and the formation of a hematoma in the tissue of the kidney or ureter. If an intermission of the oral therapy with anticoagulants with or without the use of heparin as an alternative is not possible, we avoid SWL and perform a careful ureteroscopy for stone treatment. Ureteroscopy may also bear a higher risk of bleeding in this patient group, but due to permanent visual control during the procedure, the urologist is able to avoid bleeding actively.

Treatment of patients with cardiac pacemakers are usually no problem. However, cardiology should be consulted prior to the procedure to rule out potential problems with a specific pacemaker. If the pacemaker is implanted in the abdomen, the patient should not be treated with SWL due to the risk of damaging the pacemaker.

There is no objective evidence at the moment that SWL of distal ureteral calculi in women of childbearing age has a negative effect on the ovaries or the unfertilized eggs [4]. Studies comparing spermatic function of men after SWL for distal ureteral stones and after SWL for renal or proximal ureteric stones showed reduced sperm count and motility in short term control after treatment of distal calculi. However, all parameters returned to normal values within 3 months [5]. However, there is a study showing that semen characteristics at 3 months remained lower compared to baseline, although they were within the normal range [6]. In summary, the effects of SWL on reproduction in men as well as in women are difficult to assess because many different variables have influence on fertility. Some authors are very cautious and advise women in childbearing age and men with intentions towards conception within short term after stone treatment to have no SWL procedure for distal ureteral calculi.

Preparation of the Patient

Before proceeding with the SWL procedure one has to check if the stone can be localized to target the shock wave. At the beginning of SWL in the 1980s, only ultrasound was used. This made the localization of stones in the in the middle third of the ureter almost impossible. The introduction of a dual localization system using ultrasound and fluoroscopy resulted in satisfactory localization of radiopaque calculi in the mid-ureter [7]. If a reliable localization of the stone is not possible with at least one of the two imaging modalities, the stone is not suitable for SWL. Theoretically, it would be possible to insert a ureteral catheter during cystoscopy prior to SWL and fill the ureter with contrast medium to see a radiolucent stone in the fluoroscopy image needed for SWL. However, in daily practice, this approach is too complex and one would be more likely to treat such a stone with ureteroscopy.

Positioning of the Patient Depending on the Localization of the Stone

Bone structures can impede shock waves delivered to a ureteral calculus. Therefore, the positioning of the patient has the aim to provide a direct pathway for the shockwave to travel from the skin to the stone without passing through bone. The best position of the patient depends on the location of the stone and on the type of lithotripter used.

For calculi in the proximal ureter, the shock wave may be disturbed by the transverse processes of the vertebrae. In the case of mid-ureteral or distal ureteral stones, the pelvic bones may be in the way of the shock wave.

Most proximal stones can be managed similar to renal stones with the patient in the supine position, the shock head is placed beneath the patient and is coupled to the skin dorsally. If there is interference with the transverse process of a vertebra, the shock head has to be turned to a more lateral position.

In mid-ureteral and distal calculi, the shock wave has to come from the ventral side to avoid disturbance of the shock wave by the pelvis. Using a lithotripter with the shock head always positioned underneath the patient, it is necessary to have the patient either in a "rotated supine position" or in the prone position for these cases. Some lithotripters have the possibility to rotate the shock head around to a position above the table, therefore the shock waves can be applied ventrally with the patient in supine position.

There are several papers on modifications of the supine and prone positions to increase stone free rates in specific stone localizations [8, 9]. However, any modifications depend on the stone situation of your individual patient and on the technical possibilities of your lithotripter. Proper planning prior to SWL is necessary, a CT scan performed prior to the SWL procedure may help to visualize the stone and the relevant bony structures.

Analgesia and Anesthesia

SWL can be performed with intravenous sedation or other minimal anesthetic techniques in most patients, while ureteroscopy is routinely performed under general anesthesia. Therefore, SWL is beneficial for patients who have a high risk of complications during general anesthesia or those who do not want to undergo general anesthesia for subjective reasons. However, using only analgesia or sedation during SWL, the procedure is not well-tolerated by some patients, resulting in movements of the patient during the treatment which reduces efficacy of SWL. Therefore, if a patients cannot tolerate SWL with minimal anesthetic techniques well, we advise to terminate the treatment session and to re-treat the patients under general anesthesia after accurate preparation.

Ureteral Stenting

The AUA/EAU Ureteral Stones Guidelines Panel (2007) did not recommend routine stenting of the ureter in patients undergoing SWL. Their analysis showed no improvement in stone fragmentation or passage of stone fragments when a ureteral stent was inserted. However, stent-related morbidity was found to be high when a stent was placed [1]. After ureteroscopy, the indications for ureteral stenting are ureteral injury, confirmed ureteral stricture, solitary kidney, renal insufficiency or a large residual stone burden [1].

A large systematic review on ureteral stenting during stone treatment did not show a benefit of stenting before SWL treatment of ureteral stones [10]. In a recent prospective trial, 60 patients treated with SWL for proximal ureteral stones of 2 cm or less were randomized to ureteral stenting or not prior to SWL. There was no difference between the two groups regarding stone free rate, number of treatment sessions per patient und number of shock waves delivered [11].

A meta-analysis published in 2011 found a significantly higher incidence of lower urinary symptoms after stenting before SWL compared to patients without a ureteral stent. However, there were no significant differences in regards to hematuria, fever, urinary tract infection, pain and analgesia use, nausea and vomiting or auxillary treatment between the two groups [12].

However, even after SWL or ureteroscopy without complications during operation, there may be patients who need a ureteral stent due to early or late complications: pain due to hydronephrosis caused by stone fragments or steinstrasse in the ureter, urinary tract infection in an kidney with hydronephrosis after stone treatment or ureteral stricture formation after stone treatment.

Adjunctive Medical Treatment

Selective alpha-1A-adrenergic antagonists as tamsulosin can be used to decrease the force of the ureter as alpha-adrenergic receptors, predominantly alpha-1A and alpha-1D, have been detected especially in the distal ureter. There are several trials showing better outcomes after SWL plus medical expulsive therapy (MET) with tamsulosin. A randomized controlled trial published in 2010 including 166 patients after SWL of renal calculi showed significantly improved stone free rates at

3 months after using tamsulosin and diclofenac compared to diclofenac alone (73 % versus 55 %) [13]. Another randomized controlled trial found a significant decrease in the time to stone passage in the group treated with tamsulosin compared to the placebo group [14]. A systematic review on MET after SWL by Schuler and coworkers [15] also showed a significant increase in successful outcomes [15]. In most studies, tamsulosin was administered over a longer period of time (30–90 days after SWL). Side effects of tamsulosin including decreased blood pressure or ejaculatory dysfunction were rare in these studies.

Stone Free Rates After SWL for Ureteral Calculi

According to a meta-analysis of the EAU Guidelines on Urolithiasis Panel (2012), stone free rates after primary treatment were 86 %/74 % for distal ureteral stones <10 mm/>10 mm, 84 %/76 % for mid-ureteral stones <10 mm/>10 mm and 89 %/70 % for proximal ureteral stones <10 mm/>10 mm (Table 6.1). This data shows no significant differences compared to the meta-analysis of the AUA/EAU Ureteral Stones Guidelines Panel (2007) [1, 16].

The stone free rates after primary treatment with SWL are significantly lower than the results of ureteroscopy for distal ureteral stones <10 mm and >10 mm and proximal ureteral stones >10 mm. There are no significant differences between primary treatment outcomes of SWL and ureteroscopy for mid-ureteral calculi and proximal ureteral stones <10 mm [16].

Using more than one SWL treatment session, high stone free rates of 96.1 % for proximal, 97.8 % for mid-ureteral and 97.9 % for distal ureteral calculi have been shown. Average number of SWL procedure was 1.37, 1.47 and 1.22 for proximal, mid-ureteral and distal ureteral stones [17].

Kanao et al. presented preoperative nomograms for predicting stone free rates after extracorporal shock wave lithotripsy. Stone length, stone location and number of stones were identified as independent predictors for stone clearance in their

Table 6.1 Meta-analysis of stone free rates (SFR) after primary treatment with SWL and ureteroscopy in the overall population (European Association of Urology Guidelines on Urolithiasis 2012 [16]

		SWL		Ureteroscopy	
Localization	Size (mm)	No. of patients	SFR (95 % CI)	No. of patients	SFR (95 % CI)
Distal ureter	<10	1,684	86 % (80–91)	2,013	97 % (96–98)
	>10	966	74 % (57–87)	668	93 % (91–95)
Mid ureter	<10	44	84 % (65–95)	116	93 % (88–98)
	>10	15	76 % (36–97)	110	79 % (71–87)
Proximal ureter	<10	967	89 % (87–91)	318	84 % (80–88)
	>10	481	70 % (66–74)	338	81 % (77–85)

Table 6.2 Nomograms predicting stone free rates 3 months after single SWL for solitary ureteral calculi [18]

	Length of stone (mm)				
	≤5	6–10	11–15	16–20	>20
Proximal ureter	93.8 (86–91)	86.6 (81–91)	76.4 (65–85)	56.7 (37–73)	42.2 (19–64)
Mid/distal ureter	92.3 (81–98)	83.6 (77–90)	71.8 (59–82)	51.1 (29–71)	36.9 (16–60)

% (95 % confidence interval)

analysis. The predicted stone free rates 3 months after single SWL for ureteral calculi are shown in Table 6.2 [18].

Resit-Goren and co-workers calculated the time to stone clearance after SWL for ureteral stones: Mean time to stone clearance was 2.2 days for stones <10 mm, 7.7 days for stones 11–15 mm and 12.2 days for stones >15 mm. Regarding the localization of the stone, clearance was achieved significantly faster for distal and mid-ureteral stones compared to proximal stones, however, the proximal stones were significantly larger than the stones in the two other groups and no multivariable analysis was performed. 93.1 % of all patients were stone-free 20 days after primary SWL treatment, 19.7 patients needed more than one SWL session (2–4), 6.8 % of the patients had ureteroscopy for residual calculi [19].

Parameters Influencing SWL of Ureteral Calculi

1. Technical parameters:

   - Type of lithotripter:
     The first generation lithotripter (HM3, Dornier) was developed in the 1980s [20]. Today, four generations of lithotripters are on the market. The results of studies comparing different generations of lithotripters concerning treatment of ureteral calculi are mixed. Gerber et al. compared the results of the first-generation lithotripter to a second- and a third-generation lithotripter showing higher stone-free rates with the first-generation machine [21]. In contrast, Tiselius published higher rates using two third-generation lithotripters, however, this study included no direct comparison to the HM3 [17]. Nomikos and co-workers presented a comparison of a fourth-generation lithotripter with the HM3: the demonstrated comparable results, but fewer analgesics were required using the fourth-generation machine [22]. In summary, evidence suggests that lithotripters of every generation can be used for treatment of ureteral stones with reasonable efficacy.

   - Shock rate:
     A meta-analysis of Semis and co-workers showed that outcomes of SWL with 60 shocks per minute are superior compared to 120 shocks per minute [23]. A

review by Weizer et al. and the randomized, controlled, double-blind study of Honey et al. including 163 patients with proximal ureteral stones come to the same result [24, 25].

- Energy of shock waves:
  The energy of shock waves produced by the lithotripter is proportional to the kilovoltage (kV) of the shock wave generator. The technique of voltage stepping (beginning with lower kilovoltage and stepping towards the maximum) has been shown superior compared to a fixed kilovoltage during the whole treatment: In vitro studies and clinical trials demonstrated improved stone fragmentation and less shock wave-induced damage of renal tissue [26–29].

2. Influence of stone location on mechanisms of stone fragmentation:
   Using SWL, it is more difficult to treat a stone within the ureter than within the renal pelvis or a renal calyx. The physical basics of stone fragmentation provide the explanation for this clinical observation. Four effects of SWL on stones can be distinguished [30]:

   - Compressive fracture: Shock waves generate stress of the stone which cracks mainly in areas with imperfections or defects of its molecular structure. As a result of his in vitro studies, Eisenmenger proposed a circumferential squeezing effect of shock waves on a calculus due to the fact that shock waves travel faster in stone than in water [31].
   - Spallation: Due to the change in impedance at the stone-water-interface, parts of a shock wave are reflected at the posterior surface of the stone where the wave leaves the stone. A negative pressure results which leads to tensile stress within the stone.
   - Cavitation: The shock wave creates bubbles within the water at the stone-water-interface. Collapse of these bubbles leads to disposal of energy affecting the stone.
   - Dynamic squeezing: This theory combines the squeezing and spallation hypothesis. Parts of the shock wave travel around the stone and the remaining will travel inside the calculus. The outer part travels slower than the inner part which will be also reflected at the backside of the stone. Therefore the outer part reinforces the spallation process by squeezing the stone from outside.

     All mechanisms of stone fragmentation during shock wave lithotripsy arise at the stone-water-interface. In stones impacted in the mucosa of the ureter, there is less contact of the stone surface with water. Additionally, in case of cracking of the stone, the ureteral walls may hold the fragments together not allowing them to shift.

3. Size of the stone:
   The size of a ureteral stone is an independent predictor of stone clearance after SWL as shown earlier (section on: Stone free rates after SWL for ureteral calculi).

4. Stone composition:
   SWL of calcium oxalate monohydrate stones and cystine stones are more likely to fail compared to SWL of other types of stones due to difficulties in fragmenting these stones because of their relative hardness compared to other stones. Uric acid stones may be difficult to shock as their relative radiolucency make them difficult to localize on fluoroscopy.

SWL of Ureteral Calculi in Special Stone Situations

1. Obesity:
   High body mass index can result in decreased stone free rates after SWL because the distance between skin and stone can be so large that the stone cannot be optimally brought into the focal zone of the lithotripter. According to a multivariable analysis of Perks et al., the success rate of SWL is lower when the distance between stone and skin is higher than 9 cm, independent of location and size of the calculus [32].
2. Ureteric stones in children:
   SWL can be performed in children. However, positioning of the patients may be more difficult compared to adults. The meta-analysis of the AUA/EAU Ureteral Stones Guidelines Panel (2007) showed comparable stone-free rates for children and adults in the distal and proximal ureter. In mid-ureteral stones, clearance rates were even higher in the pediatric population compared with adults [1]. However, the data for SWL in the pediatric patient must be interpreted cautiously as it is based on studies with small numbers of patients. A randomized, controlled trial of Basiri and co-workers with 50 children randomized to SWL and 50 randomized to ureteroscopy showed that both procedures were feasible in experienced hands in children at the age of 1–13 years with distal ureteral stones. However, efficacy rates were higher in the ureteroscopy group. Two patients sustained ureteral perforation during ureteroscopy, other complications in both groups were minor [33]. In our opinion, the small size of urethra und ureter in young children favors SWL as primary treatment in children with ureteral stones.

Complications of SWL

According to the AUA/EAU Ureteral Stones Guidelines Panel (2007), the most frequent complications of SWL for ureteral stones are steinstrasse with or without hydronephrosis, urinary tract infection, sepsis, ureteral injury and ureteral stricture formation. Median complication rates showed no significant difference between stones in the distal, mid or proximal ureter. Steinstrasse is a typical complication of SWL which is not seen after ureteroscopy. The rates of ureteral injuries and strictures are slightly higher after ureteroscopy compared to SWL. The rates of urinary tract infections and sepsis are similar for both treatment modalities. Serious complications such as loss of kidney function, significant ureteral/renal hematomy, loss of a kidney and death are rare and thus their incidence is difficult to report [1].

Take Home Points

- SWL and ureteroscopy are first line treatment options for patients with ureteral calculi. Prior to undergoing treatment of their ureteral stone, patients should be informed about the advantages and disadvantages of both procedures.
- Contraindications to SWL for the treatment of ureteral calculi include pregnancy, untreated urinary tract infections, untreated coagulopathy, and large aortic aneurysms.
- The stone free rates after primary treatment with SWL are significantly lower than the results of ureteroscopy for distal ureteral stones <10 mm and >10 mm and proximal ureteral stones >10 mm. There are no significant differences between primary treatment outcomes of SWL and ureteroscopy for mid-ureteral calculi and proximal ureteral stones <10 mm [16]
- Adjunctive medical treatment with tamsulosin increases stone free rates after SWL. Routine stenting of the ureter is not necessary prior to SWL for most stones.

References

1. Preminger GM, Tiselius HG, Assimos DG, Alken P, Buck AC, Gallucci M, Knoll T, Lingeman JE, Nakada SY, Pearle MS, Sarica K, Türk C, Wolf Jr JS. 2007 guideline for the management of ureteral calculi. Eur Urol. 2007;52:1610–31.
2. Hruza M, Schulze M, Teber D, Goezen AS, Rassweiler J. Laparoscopic techniques for removal of renal and ureteral calculi. J Endourol. 2009;23:1713–8.
3. Rassweiler J, Lutz K, Gumpinger R, Eisenberger F. Efficacy of in situ extracorporeal shock wave lithotripsy for upper ureteral calculi. Eur Urol. 1986;12:377–86.
4. Vieweg J, Weber HM, Miller K, Hautmann R. Female fertility following extracorporal shock wave lithotripsy of distal ureteral calculi. J Urol. 1992;148:1007.
5. Martinez Portillo FJ, Heidenreich A, Schwarzer U, Michel MS, Alken P, Engelmann U. Microscopic and biochemical fertility characteristics of semen after shock wave lithotripsy of distal ureteral calculi. J Endourol. 2001;15:781–4; discussion 784–5.
6. Bedir S, Kilciler M, Cincik M, Ozgok Y. Relationship between extracorporal shock wave lithotripsy and semen parameters in patients with lower ureteral stones. Fertil Steril. 2004;82:1687–8.
7. Rassweiler J, Henkel TO, Joyce A, Köhrmann KU, Manning M, Alken P. Extracorporeal shock wave lithotripsy of ureteric stones with the Modulith SL 20. BJU. 1992;70:594–9.
8. Kose AC, Demirbas M. The modified prone position: a new approach for treating pre-vesical stones with extracorporal shock wave lithotripsy. BJU Int. 2004;93:369–73.
9. Hara N, Koike H, Bilim V, Takahashi K, Nishiyama T. Efficacy of extracorporal shock wave lithotripsy with patients in rotated spine or rotated prone for treating ureteral stones: a case-control study. J Endourol. 2006;20:170–4.
10. Haleblian G, Kijvikai K, de la Rosette J, Preminger G. Ureteral stenting and urinary stone management: a systematic review. J Urol. 2008;179:424–30.
11. Ghoneim IA, El-Ghoneimy MN, El-Naggar AE, Hammoud KM, El-Gammal MY, Morsi AA. Extracorporal shock wave lithotripsy in impacted upper ureteral stones: a prospective randomized comparison between stented and non-stented techniques. Urology. 2010;75:45–50.

12. Pengfei S, Min J, Jie Y, Xiong L, Wuran W, Yi D, Hao Z, Jia W. Use of ureteral stent in extracorporal shock wave lithotripsy for upper urinary calculi: a systematic review and meta-analysis. J Urol. 2011;186:1328–35.
13. Hussein M. Does tamsulosin increase stone clearance after shock wave lithotripsy of renal stones? A prospective, randomized controlled study. Scand J Urol Nephrol. 2010;44:27–31.
14. Falahatkar S, Kgosropanah I, Vajary AD, Bateni ZH, Khosropanah D, Allahkhah A. Is there a role for tamsulosin after shock wave lithotripsy in the treatment of renal and ureteral calculi? J Endourol. 2011;25:495–8.
15. Schuler TD, Shahani R, Honey RJ, Pace KT. Medical expulsive therapy as an adjunct to improve shock wave lithotripsy outcomes: a systematic review and meta-analysis. J Endourol. 2009;23:387–93.
16. Türk C, Knoll T, Petrik A, Sarica K, Straub M, Seitz C. European association of urology guidelines on urolithiasis. EAU Guidelines, edition presented at the EAU Annual Congress Milan 2013. ISBN 978-90-79754-71-7.
17. Tiselius H-G. How efficient is extracorporal shockwave lithotripsy with modern lithotripters for removal of ureteral stones? J Endourol. 2008;22:249–55.
18. Kanao K, Nakashima J, Nakagawa K, Asakura H, Miyajima A, Oya M, Ohigashi T, Murai M. Preoperative nomograms for predicting stone free rate after extracorporal shock wave lithotripsy. J Urol. 2006;176:1453–7.
19. Resit-Goren M, Dirim A, Ilteris-Tekin M, Ozkardes H. Time to stone clearance for ureteral stones treated with extracorporal shock wave lithotripsy. Urology. 2011;78:26–31.
20. Fuchs G, Miller K, Rassweiler J, Eisenberger F. Extracorporeal shock wave lithotripsy: one-year experience with the Dornier lithotripter. Eur Urol. 1985;11:145–9.
21. Gerber R, Studer UE, Danuser H. Is new always better? A comparative study of three lithotripter generations. J Urol. 2005;173:2013–6.
22. Nomikos MS, Sowter SJ, Tolley DA. Outcomes using a fourth-generation lithotripter: a new benchmark for comparison? BJU Int. 2007;100:1356–60.
23. Semins MJ, Trock BJ, Matlaga BR. The effect of shock wave rate on the outcome of shock wave lithotripsy: a meta-analysis. J Urol. 2008;179:194–7; discussion 197.
24. Weizer AZ, Zhong P, Preminger GM. New concepts in shock wave lithotripsy. Urol Clin North Am. 2002;34:375–82.
25. Honey RJD`A, Schuler TD, Ghiculete D, Pace KT, Canadian Endourology Group. A randomized, double-blind trial to compare shock wave frequencies of 60 and 120 shocks per minute for upper ureteral stones. J Urol. 2009;182:1418–23.
26. Zhou Y, Cocks FH, Preminger GM, Zhong P. The effect of treatment strategy on stone comminution efficiency in shock wave lithotripsy. J Urol. 2004;172:349–54.
27. Connors BA, Evvan AP, Blomgren PM, Handa RK, Willis LR, Gao S. Effect of initial shock wave voltage on shock wave lithotripsy-induced lesion size during step-wise voltage ramping. BJU Int. 2008;103:104–7.
28. Demirci D, Sofikerim M, Yalcin E, Ekmekcioglu O, Gülmez I, Karacagil M. Comparison of conventional and step-wise shock wave lithotripsy in management of urinary calculi. J Endourol. 2007;21:1407–10.
29. Lambert EH, Walsh R, Moreno MW, Gupta M. Effect of escalating versus fixed voltage treatment on stone comminution and renal injury during extracorporeal shock wave lithotripsy: a prospective randomized trial. J Urol. 2010;183:580–4.
30. Rassweiler JJ, Knoll T, Köhrmann KU, McAteer JA, Cleveland RO, Bailey MR, Chaussy C. Shock wave technology and application: an update. Eur Urol. 2011;59:784–96.
31. Eisenmenger W. The mechanisms of stone fragmentation in ESWL. Ultrasound Med Biol. 2001;27:683–93.
32. Perks AE, Schuler TD, Lee J, Ghiculete D, Chung DG, Honey RJD´A, Pace KT. Stone attenuation and skin-to-stone distance on computed tomography predicts for stone fragmentation by shock wave lithotripsy. Urology. 2008;72:765–9.
33. Basiri A, Zare S, Tabibi A, Sharifiaghdas F, Aminsharifi A, Mousavi-Bahar SH, Ahmadnia H. A multicenter, randomized, controlled trial of transurethral and shock wave lithotripsy – which is the best minimally invasive modality to treat distal ureteral calculi in children? J Urol. 2010;184:1106–10.

Chapter 7
Semirigid Ureteroscopy for Ureteral Calculi

Michael Maddox, Mary Powers, and Raju Thomas

Introduction

There has been a considerable paradigm shift in the management of nephrolithiasis, with increasing concentration on minimally invasive treatment options. Ureteroscopy remains a mainstay in the treatment of urolithiasis, and patients and urologists alike have benefited from significant technologic advancements in ureteroscopic equipment over the past three decades.

Given the familiarity of endoscopic procedures, it is not surprising that urologists have adopted rigid ureteroscopy as essentially an extension of cystoscopy. In fact, Young was the first to report on ureteroscopy in 1912, which was performed with a pediatric cystoscope [1]. Since that time, ureteroscopes have evolved from rigid to semirigid and finally to flexible scopes in order to improve ureteral and renal access while limiting the morbidity of ureteroscopic procedures.

Initial experience with rigid ureteroscopes involved a 13 French (Fr) diameter scope, which utilized a rod-lens system and was pioneered by Richard Wolf Medical Instruments [2]. A major limitation of this scope was the inability to bend the scope without distorting the visibility or damaging the optics mechanism. This was modified by ACMI's Rigiflex scope in 1985 with the introduction of fiberoptics, creating the first semirigid ureteroscope capable of navigating the tortuous course of the ureter with better visibility [3]. Improving on this design was Candela Laser Corporation's downsizing of the scope, known as a "miniscope" with two independent working channels [4]. Continued improvements on this theme have led to contemporary semirigid ureteroscopes, as well as flexible scopes and digital endoscopes affording drastically improved image quality. This in turn has directly contributed to safer application of this equipment with better outcomes.

M. Maddox (✉) • M. Powers • R. Thomas
Department of Urology, Tulane University School of Medicine, New Orleans, LA, USA
e-mail: mmaddox2@tulane.edu; mpowers1@tulane.edu; rthomas@tulane.edu

S.R. Patel, S.Y. Nakada (eds.), *Ureteral Stone Management: A Practical Approach*, DOI 10.1007/978-3-319-08792-4_7

Indications for Semirigid Ureteroscopy

Ureteroscopy is the use of an endoscope that can be passed through the lower urogenital tract into the ureter. It serves many purposes, including both diagnostic and therapeutic. Typically performed under general anesthesia, ureteroscopy allows a less invasive approach to treatment of numerous conditions including calculi, strictures or tumors. Contemporary ureteroscopy is dichotomized based on the instruments being employed into flexible and semirigid. Newer flexible ureteroscopy allows better visualization of the renal collecting system (particularly the lower pole) and can gain access to ureters that do not accommodate the semi-rigid ureteroscope. However, semirigid ureteroscopy (SRURS) is a long-standing surgical technique with a variety of indications as well as advantages over its flexible counterpart.

The most common use for SRURS is for the treatment of ureteral calculi. The endoscope can be passed into the bladder through the urethra and then to cannulate the ureteral orifice. While the narrowest portions of the ureter to traverse include the ureterovesical junction, the ureteric crossing of the iliac vessels or the ureteropelvic junction, SRURS is often successful at reaching the upper ureter. This in conjunction with its working channels facilitates either stone basket extraction or holmium laser lithotripsy of ureteral calculi. Using the working channel of the ureteroscope, basket extractors, laser fibers, and pneumatic lithotripters can aid in stone management.

The size of the ureteral or renal calculi must be taken into account. If a patient has persistent renal colic due to ureteral calculi after a trial of spontaneous passage, these calculi can be managed endoscopically. Typically stones <10 mm in diameter can be safely managed via retrograde endoscopy with SRURS. Location of the stone is also a factor as the success of SRURS or ureteroscopy in general can vary based on the location, which is discussed later in the chapter [5].

Ureteral strictures can result from stone disease, prolonged indwelling ureteral stents, or from iatrogenic causes. Ureteroscopic manipulation carries a small risk of stricture occurrence itself. However, SRURS can also be used in stricture management to facilitate laser endoureterotomy, endopyelotomy or balloon dilation [6].

Ureteral transitional cell carcinoma (TCC) represents a minority of the total cases of transitional cell carcinoma. Of those cases of ureteral TCC, the distal, mid and proximal ureter experience a frequency of 73, 24, and 3 % respectively in cancer occurrence [7]. Diagnosis of these tumors can be performed by SRURS as well as for treatment. Small volume, low-grade ureteral tumors can be biopsied as well as fulgurated or ablated using SRURS. Surveillance of the upper tracts can also be performed.

Flank pain secondary to renal colic is the most common cause of abdominal pain in pregnant patients unrelated to gynecologic problems [5]. Typically ultrasonography is performed to reduce radiation exposure although IVP, CT and MRI are alternative modalities to evaluate for ureteral calculi. Ulvik et al. reported good success rates in ureteroscopic stone removal in pregnant patients without the need for temporizing internal stents or nephrostomy tubes [8]. Similar studies have shown that ureteroscopy has low morbidity to the patient with minimal risk of fetal injury [5].

Another population that may benefit from SRURS are those patients with either bleeding diatheses or those who are not able to stop anti-coagulation due to other medical comorbidities. Watterson et al. demonstrated the safety as well as efficacy of using small caliber ureteroscopes with holmium laser lithotripsy to treat upper tract stones in such a population [9].

The pediatric population can also benefit from SRURS. While children seem to be more successful in stone passage from extracorporeal shockwave lithotripsy, SRURS can be used as a primary treatment or as a second line treatment for ESWL failure [10]. SRURS can be of particular benefit in patients with anatomic abnormalities or specifically hard stones such as brushite or cystine. Smaller ureteroscopes are available in 4.5 and 6.0 Fr to utilize in ureteroscopic manipulation. Adult sized ureteroscopes can also be used to evaluate the bladder if a pediatric cystoscope is unavailable.

Other more rare uses of SRURS include ureteroscopic ureteral realignment in a transected ureter. With combination use of antegrade flexible ureteroscopy and retrograde semirigid ureteroscopy Liu et al. were able to successfully realign the ureters of eight patients in whom iatrogenic injury had been noted in the immediate postoperative period [11]. SRURS can also be of use in the removal or relocation of migrated stents that no longer demonstrate a distal curl in the bladder but rather in the ureter. We will focus in this chapter on the use of semirigid ureteroscopy in the management of ureteral calculi.

Technique

Performing semirigid ureteroscopy should be done systematically with care to prevent any complication or injury. Essential to ensure that semirigid ureteroscopy is performed safely is an awareness of the tortuous ureteral anatomy, proximity of surrounding structures (particularly the iliac vessels), and segments that are inherently more susceptible to injury. Patient specific information should be reviewed including preoperative imaging studies with attention to any evidence of potential stone impaction as well as stone size and location. Additionally, all patients should have sterile urine prior to ureteroscopic manipulation to reduce the risk of sepsis.

Although the endoscopic armamentarium available to urologists today has vastly expanded since ureteroscopy was first described, there is some equipment that is universally essential to successful ureteroscopy. The standard rigid and flexible cystoscopy sets should be available in addition to a variety of guide-wires, a ureteral catheter, balloon dilator, ureteral stents, as well as working instruments for stone treatment including a Holmium laser and fiber and stone baskets. A typical set up for semirigid ureteroscopy is seen in Fig. 7.1.

Room set up should mimic that of cystoscopy with ergonomic placement of video and fluoroscopic monitors. Normal saline is the preferred irrigation solution to limit adverse events as a result of potential systemic absorption during ureteroscopy. Pressure irrigation may improve visibility and most commonly is achieved

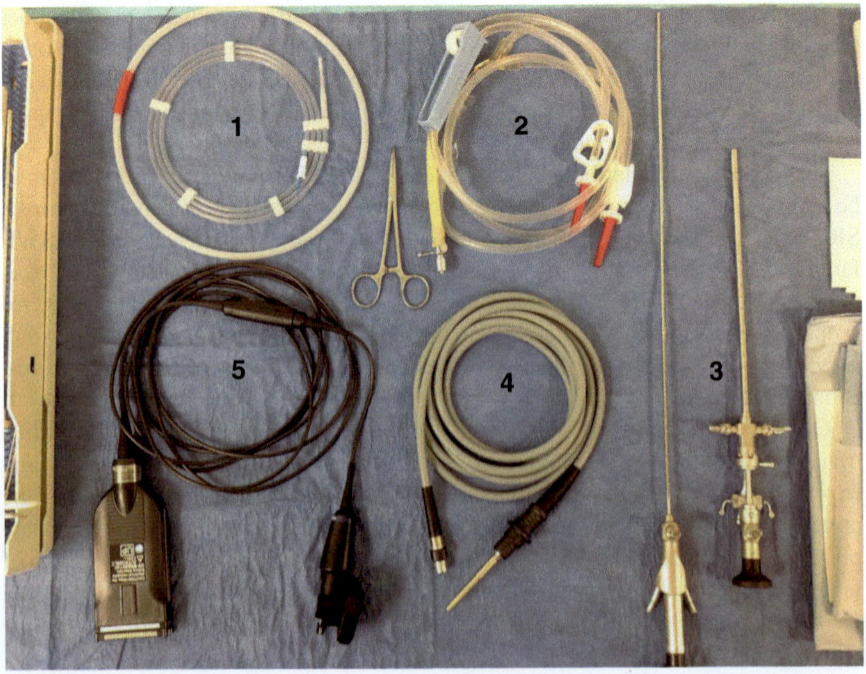

Fig. 7.1 Table set-up for SRURS: *1* Guide wires, *2* Irrigation tubing, *3* Cystoscope and semirigid ureteroscope, *4* Light cord, *5* Video camera (*clockwise from top left*)

with a pressure bag or hand-help pump syringe. A Level 1 System can also be used to control irrigation as well as to warm the irrigant to body temperature (Level NORMOFLO Irrigation Warming Set, Smiths Medical ASD, Rockland, MA, USA).

Cystoscopy is performed as an initial step to every ureteroscopy to rule out incidental bladder pathology and facilitate passage of the guide-wire into the ureter using fluoroscopy. We prefer to perform semirigid ureteroscopy along side a stiff guide wire such as an Amplatz Super Stiff™ wire (Boston Scientific, Natick, MA). A stiff wire has the potential benefit of straightening the course of the ureter, which is particularly useful in men with a large prostate and J-hook in the distal ureter or those with previous reimplants creating a distorted course of the distal ureter. This should however be exchanged after a floppy tipped guide-wire such as a Bentson™ wire (Cook Medical, Bloomington, IN) is placed into the ureter to limit the possibility of ureteral trauma/perforation.

Once access to the ureter is gained by passage of a guide-wire, this access should remain intact as a safety measure until the ureteroscopy procedure is completed. The guide-wire should be secured to the contralateral drape with a hemostat, which will prevent migration or inadvertent removal.

Passage of the semirigid ureteroscope should be performed with considerable caution as the tip of the scope can easily create false passages in the urethra or distal ureter. This is particularly true in the male urethra as the external sphincter

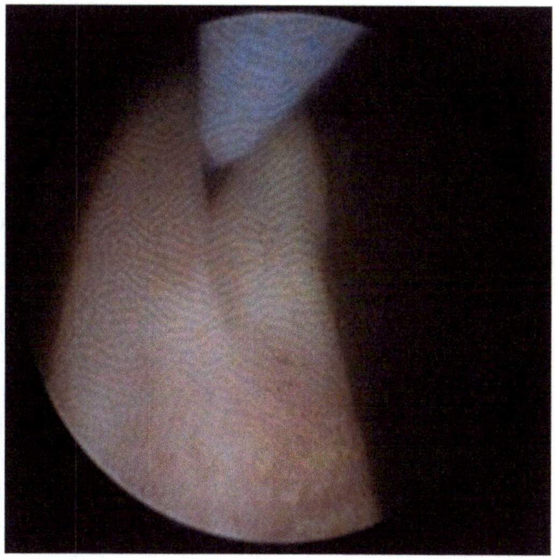

Fig. 7.2 Attempting to insert semirigid ureteroscope into right ureteral orifice below guide wire

and prostate can act as a fulcrum. It is imperative that the urethral and ureteral lumen be maintained in the center of the visual field to minimize the possibility of a false passage.

Upon entry into the bladder, the ureteral orifice is located and the scope is passed underneath the previously placed guide-wire. This maneuver facilitates passage of the scope into the distal ureter utilizing the guide-wire to open the ureteral orifice. This maneuver is demonstrated in Fig. 7.2. Occasionally, passing a second guide-wire under direct vision through the working channel of the ureteroscope can facilitate traversing the ureteral orifice. Additionally, using pressurized irrigation may also help with passage of the scope into the ureteral orifice. However, when performing SRURS for the treatment of stones, the surgeon must be cognizant of the possibility of proximal migration of the stone as a result of the pressurized irrigation. If resistance is met during passage of the ureteroscope at any point during the procedure, the safety of proceeding should be weighed against the risk of potential complications.

Although some caution against use of the semirigid ureteroscope for procedures proximal to the iliac vessels, advances in technology of the semirigid scopes can allow for safe passage into the proximal ureter in many patients. Obstacles to proximal ureteroscopy with the semirigid scope include large muscular habitus (presumably due to large psoas muscles), previous ureteral surgery, and obesity. If difficulties are encountered under these clinical settings, consideration of flexible ureteroscopy as an alternative must be exercised.

In the management of ureteral stones with semirigid ureteroscopy, there are a variety of treatment options. Among the instruments in the armamentarium of most urologists performing SRURS are various stone baskets, Holmium: YAG lasers of different diameters, as well as pneumatic and electrohydraulic (EHL) lithotripters. However, Holmium: YAG lasers have emerged as the standard of care in contemporary endoscopic lithotripsy. Reasons for laser lithotripsy are primarily related to improved efficacy and safety profiles.

Holmium lasers are not limited by stone composition, as they are effective in fragmenting all stone types. In addition, compared to EHL and pneumatic devices, the holmium laser produces smaller stone fragments during lithotripsy [12]. The holmium laser safety profile is significantly better than EHL as the laser energy is absorbed in the fluid medium of ureteroscopy and thus can safely be activated at a distance of 0.5–9 mm without the risk of ureteral injury or perforation [13].

Laser lithotripsy may be performed utilizing two different techniques depending on the stone size and characteristics. For the smaller stone, it is beneficial to "paint" or "dust" the stone with the laser fiber, essentially removing the outer borders of the stone as dust fragments. This can be done to completion, or if preferred, the stone may be reduced in size using this technique until amenable to stone basketing the fragments of the stone. In the setting of larger stones or impacted ureteral stones, the ureteral stone is typically fragmented into several pieces by using the laser to split the stones into halves. Once this is achieved, either the stones may be basketed or further fragmented using the "paint" technique.

There are a number of stone retrieval devices available for removal of stones or stone fragments during ureteroscopy. Many of these devices are Nitinol-based stone baskets, which are our preferred stone retrieval device. There are many variations of these devices, which are primarily tipless baskets or grasping devices, which combine the abilities of conventional stone baskets with those of three-prong graspers. These stone retrieval devices are discussed in more detail elsewhere in this book.

Whether it is necessary to leave a stent following semirigid ureteroscopy is a matter of some debate. At our institution, this decision is determined by individual surgeon preference, and characteristics of the patient and ease of the procedure weigh heavily on the ultimate decision to use a ureteral stent. There is level one evidence to support that after uncomplicated semirigid ureteroscopy, there is no benefit to ureteral stent placement. In fact, much of the literature demonstrates an increased incidence and severity of postoperative pain, increased analgesic use, and bothersome voiding symptoms in those patients who are stented following ureteroscopy [14, 15].

Tips and Tricks of Semirigid Ureteroscopy

In the event of difficult access to the ureter, there are a number of potential tricks that may aid in the passage of the ureteroscope [16]. One such technique involves the use of an additional guide-wire through a working channel of the ureteroscope. This "railroad" technique may enable the ureteroscope to be more precisely guided into the distal ureter and facilitate passage of the scope as seen in Fig. 7.3. This may be of particular use when manipulating the ureteroscope proximal to the iliac vessels, and may overcome some patient-specific anatomical challenges such as the large psoas muscle mentioned previously.

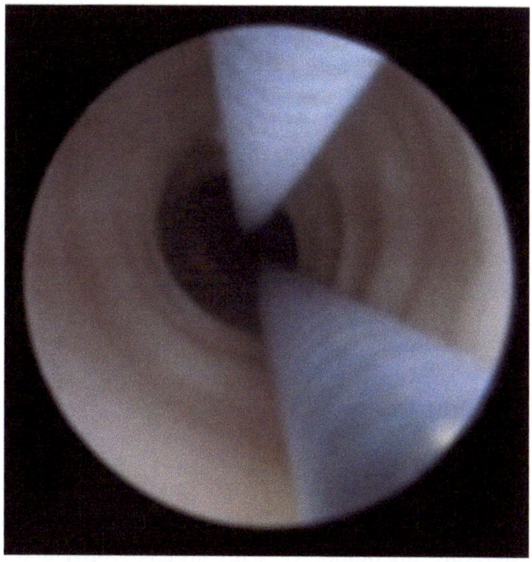

Fig. 7.3 The railroad technique: one guide wire is seen adjacent to the SRURs. The second guide wire is inserted through the working channel of the ureteroscope, mimicking a "railroad track"

Another technique, particularly in females and children, is the use of serial fascial dilators up to 10Fr passed over a guide-wire under fluoroscopic guidance in order to dilate the ureteral orifice. The fascial dilators are inexpensive and have a good balance of tip flexibility as well as rigidity to safely dilate the ureteral orifice. In the male patient, it is our experience that the use of a balloon dilator is the preferred and safest method for dilating the ureteral orifice. This can be done either under fluoroscopy, direct vision, or a combination of the two. If either of these techniques does not allow passage of the scope, one may consider passage of a ureteral stent to allow for passive dilation and return for ureteroscopy at a later date.

Occasionally poor visualization is an issue when performing SRURS. In this event, any instrument within the working channel of the ureteroscope should be removed to identify this as an impediment to the inflow of irrigation. If this is not the source of the poor visibility, ensure that the scope is not bent using fluoroscopy, which may limit the irrigation potential. Irrigation with the use of a pressurized bag may be utilized to help improve visibility within the ureter, and this practice is our preferred method during ureteroscopy. Alternatively, an assistant may use the Single Action Pumping System™ (Boston Scientific, Natick, MA). This gives the surgeon control of the irrigation pressure and can be used when needed. When utilizing pressurized irrigation, the surgeon should be cognizant of the potential for ureteral stone migration as well as pyelovenous backflow, and therefore, the least amount of pressure necessary should be employed.

In the event of impacted stones, it may be difficult to gain access to the more proximal ureteral segment with the guide-wire. In this circumstance, our algorithm typically involves passage of a 5Fr ureteral catheter just distal to the stone. We then use an angled GlideWire to gently attempt traversing the impacted stone. If this is unsuccessful, one may inject some viscous lidocaine through the ureteral catheter in an attempt to lubricate the ureter in order to facilitate passage of the guide-wire.

Occasionally a stone may be grasped using a ureteral stone basket device without the ability to subsequently remove the stone or dislodge the stone from the basket. In this circumstance, the surgeon should disassemble the basket extracorporeally, which usually allows for removal of the basket after dislodging the stone from the basket. In the event that this is unsuccessful, the disassembled basket should be left within the ureter and the scope removed carefully. Subsequently, the semirigid ureteroscope may be passed alongside the basket and a laser fiber can be used to fragment the stone lodged within the basket. This should facilitate removal of the stone basketing device and hopefully the stone fragments.

Outcomes

Efficacy of semirigid ureteroscopy is measured by complete treatment of urolithiasis in the absence of adverse events. Non-uniform reporting plagues the urologic literature on outcomes with ureteroscopy, and thus conclusions drawn from the available series should be interpreted with some caution or at least awareness of the considerable heterogeneity of procedure and patient characteristics. In addition, the success of ureteroscopy varies considerably with respect to stone size and location, stone composition, type of ureteroscope used (semirigid versus flexible or a combination), lithotripter (laser, electrohydraulic, pneumatic), and surgeon experience. We discuss the available stone-free rates reported in contemporary literature.

In 791 semirigid procedures, El-Nahas et al. achieved a stone-free rate (SFR) of 87 % after a single operation for ureteral stones. Using a multivariate analysis, proximal ureteral location, stone impaction, stone width, and surgeon experience were independent predictors of unfavorable results (defined as residual stone or complication with the procedure) [17]. In a prospective, randomized trial of shock wave lithotripsy versus ureteroscopy for distal ureteral calculi, 29 of 32 patients in the semirigid ureteroscopy cohort were rendered stone free (90.6 %), with the remaining three patients being asymptomatic but without radiographic assessment of stone treatment efficacy [18]. Using a pneumatic lithotripter and semirigid ureteroscope, Aghamir et al. found an overall SFR of 89.5 % in 362 procedures with a mean stone size of 10.4 mm. However, the analysis included distal, mid, and proximal ureteral stones of all sizes with significant variation of success based on size and location, with the highest success rates being seen with distal stones less than 10 mm (97.4 %) [19]. Similarly, Sozen et al. reported on 500 patients undergoing SRURS for ureteral stones regardless of location. They quote an overall SFR of 94.6 %, with improved results with smaller stones (<10 mm 97.1 % versus >10 mm 83.7 % SFR) [20].

Although SFRs may be enhanced with the use of flexible ureteroscopes, Wu et al. demonstrated the feasibility of SRURS alone in the treatment of proximal ureteral stones, with a SFR of 83.2 %. When these stones were broken down into <10 mm and >10 mm, SFRs were 91.1 and 76.8 % respectively [21]. Using semirigid ureteroscopy for larger proximal ureteral stones (mean 18.5 mm), SFR was diminished considerably to 35 % demonstrating the impact of patient characteristics on successful outcomes [22].

When pooling the results of semirigid and flexible ureteroscopy, there is generally an improvement in reported overall SFR. With a mean stone size of 11.3 mm in 598 patients, use of SRURS below the iliac vessels and flexible ureteroscopy proximal to this, there was an overall SFR of 97 % in one series [23]. In a similar study focused on only proximal ureteral stones, 32 patients with a mean stone size of 8.3 mm were rendered stone-free in 96.8 % of cases using both flexible and semirigid ureteroscopy [24].

The Clinical Research Office of the Endourological Society (CROES) prospectively collected data on 9,681 patients undergoing ureteroscopic stone treatment in the Ureteroscopy Global Study. Stone free rates for distal, mid, and proximal ureteral stones were 94.2, 89.4, and 84.5 % respectively [25]. In a similar collective effort, the European Association of Urology and American Urological Association updated their guidelines on the management of ureteral calculi. Using pooled data of all ureteroscopy techniques via a meta-analysis, overall SFRs (independent of stone size) for distal, mid and proximal ureteral stones were 94, 86, and 81 % respectively [5]. Although success may vary based on stone size, location and experience among other parameters, semirigid ureteroscopy offers excellent stone free rates when used in the treatment of ureteral calculi. A summary of the above-mentioned studies is shown in Table 7.1.

Complications

Contemporary ureteroscopy has imparted improved patient safety with the advent of smaller caliber scopes with improved optics, digital ureteroscopes, holmium lasers for intracorporeal lithotripsy, and advances in adjunct instruments such as nitinol stone baskets. Despite these advances however, semirigid ureteroscopy carries inherent risk of complications that can vary from minor to more complex problems. Inability to start the procedure can occur when benign prostatic hyperplasia or other abnormal anatomy distorts the trigone making cannulation of the ureteral orifice difficult or in some cases impossible. Similarly, stenotic ureteral openings may require ureteral dilation or placement of a ureteral stent with delayed ureteroscopic intervention.

Complications can be classified as immediate or intraoperative, perioperative, or delayed. Ureteral injury is the most obvious intraoperative complication encountered with semirigid ureteroscopy. Iatrogenic ureteral injury can range on a spectrum from mucosal abrasion to false passage or ureteral perforation. The most severe manifestation of ureteral injury is complete disruption and intussusception of the ureter, which can occur with aggressive stone basketing or proceeding with ureteroscopy despite identification of a more minor ureteral injury.

SRURS can result in de novo renal obstruction with postoperative edema from instrumentation or ureteral stricture formation. Conversely, new onset of vesicoureteral reflux has also been described [26]. Postoperative obstruction and ultimately renal function deterioration is the primary concern, and it is generally our practice

Table 7.1 Stone-free rates in previously published series

Series	Patients/procedures	Stone location (%)		Stone size		Type of ureteroscope	Stone free rate	
El-Nahes [17]	791	Upper	N/A	12 mm		Semi rigid	87 %	
		Middle	N/A					
		Lower	N/A					
Pearle [18]	32	Lower	100 %	6.4 mm		Semi rigid	90.6 %	
Aghamir [19]	362	Upper	32 %	10.4 mm		Semi rigid	<10 mm	91.7 %
		Middle	17 %				>10 mm	85.8 %
		Lower	51 %				Overall	89.5 %
Sozen [20]	500	Upper	7.2 %	Upper	7.36 mm	Semi rigid and flexible	<10 mm	97.1 %
		Middle	9.4 %	Middle	9.06 mm		>10 mm	83.7 %
		Lower	83.4 %	Lower	8.77 mm		Overall	94.6 %
Wu [21]	101	Upper	100 %	<10 mm	7.2 mm	Semi rigid	<10 mm	91.1 %
				>10 mm	17 mm		>10 mm	76.8 %
				Overall	12.6 mm		Overall	83.2 %
Lee [22]	42	Upper	100 %	18.5 mm		Semi rigid	35 %	
Sofer [23]	598	Upper	32.4 %	11.3 mm		Semi rigid and flexible	Renal	84 %
		Middle	18.6 %				Upper	97 %
		Lower	39.6 %				Middle	100 %
		Renal	9.4 %				Lower	98 %
							Overall	97 %

Lam [24]	31	Upper	100 %	8.2 mm	Semi rigid and flexible	<10 mm	100 %
						>10 mm	93 %
						Overall	96.8 %
Castro [25]	9,555	Upper	27.8 %	NA	Semi rigid and flexible	Upper	84.5 %
		Middle	20.7 %			Middle	89.4 %
		Lower	46.9 %			Lower	94.2 %
		Multiple	4.6 %			Multiple	76.6 %
Preminger [5]	15,016	Upper	42.8 %	NA	Semi rigid and flexible	Upper	81 %
		Middle	10.7 %			Middle	86 %
		Lower	46.5 %			Lower	94 %

NA not available

Table 7.2 Complication rates based on location of ureteral stone after URS [5, 26, 28, 29]

	Proximal ureter (%)	Middle ureter	Distal ureter
Sepsis	4	4	2
Steinstrasse	0		
Stricture	2	4	1
Ureteral injury	6	6	3
UTI	4	2	4
Subcapsular hematoma	0.36	0	0

to selectively obtain a renal ultrasound 4–6 weeks following ureteroscopy to ensure there is no silent obstructive process that can compromise renal function.

Infectious complications are among the most commonly encountered following semirigid ureteroscopy. Stone culture has superior predictive value of post-operative systemic inflammatory response syndrome compared to bladder urine culture following upper tract stone surgery [27]. Unfortunately, this information is rarely available prior to surgery and thus semirigid ureteroscopy with stone manipulation can lead to urinary tract infections, or more severely, to sepsis. Schuster et al. reported a UTI rate of 1 % and sepsis rate of 0.3 % [26]. Other studies give ranges of 2–4 % for UTI or sepsis as seen in Table 7.2.

More rare complications of SRURS include steinstrasse ("stone street"), when stone fragments block the ureter leading to obstruction. Renal hematoma after ureteroscopy can also occur. Chiu et al. evaluated over 1,000 patients who underwent ureteroscopy and found a subcapsular hematoma in 0.36 % of patients [28]. Flank pain, fever and dropping hemoglobin were the presenting symptoms and more commonly occurred in patients with thin cortical parenchyma. Other uncommon complications include clot retention, urinary extravasation or retroperitoneal fibrosis [26, 29].

Take-Home Points

- Semirigid ureteroscopy can be used with great success rates for the treatment of ureteral calculi.
- Stone free rates vary depending on stone size and location, but in general, with experience, the SFR exceeds 80 % regardless of location and size with semirigid ureteroscopy.
- Semirigid ureteroscopy has proven to be a safe procedure in the treatment of stone disease with acceptably low complication rates.
- Directed perioperative antibiotics should be employed in all cases complicit with guideline recommendations in order to limit the occurrence of infectious complications.
- In the event of an iatrogenic ureteral injury, the procedure should be aborted and a stent should be placed if possible, in order to prevent more severe injury.

References

1. Young HH, McKay RW. Congenital valvular obstruction of the prostatic urethra. Surg Gynecol Obstet. 1929;48:509.
2. Bagley DH. Ureteroscopy. AUA Update Series. 1994;13:206.
3. Payne DA, Keeley Jr FX, et al. Rigid and flexible ureteroscopes: technical features. In: Smith AD, Badlani GH, Preminger GM, editors. Smith's textbook of endourology. 3rd ed. Hoboken: Wiley-Blackwell; 2012. p. 365–87. Ch 34.
4. Dretler SP, Cho G. Semirigid ureteroscopy: a new genre. J Urol. 1989;141:1314–6.
5. Preminger G, Tiselius HG, Assimos D, et al. 2007 Guideline for management of ureteral calculi. J Urol. 2007;178:2418–34.
6. Mendez-Torres FR, Urena R, Thomas R. Retrograde ureteroscopic endopyelotomy. Urol Clin N Am. 2004;31(1):99–106.
7. Vikram R, Sandler CM, Ng CS. Imaging and staging of transitional cell carcinoma: part 2, upper urinary tract. AJR Am J Roentgenol. 2009;192(6):1488–93.
8. Ulvik NM, Bakke A, Hoisaeter PA. Ureteroscopy in pregnancy. J Urol. 1995;154:1660–3.
9. Watterson JD, Girvan AR, Cook AJ, et al. Safety and efficacy of holmium: YAG laser lithotripsy in patients with bleeding diatheses. J Urol. 2002;168:442–5.
10. Thomas R, Ortenberg J, Lee BR, et al. Safety and efficacy of pediatric ureteroscopy for management of calculous disease. J Urol. 1993;149:1082–4.
11. Liu C, Zhang X, Xue D, et al. Endoscopic realignment in the management of the complete transected ureter. Int Urol Nephrol. 2014;46:335–40.
12. Teichman JM, Vassar GJ, Bishoff JT, et al. Holmium: YAG lithotripsy yields smaller fragments than Lithoclast, pulsed dye laser, or electrohydraulic lithotripsy. J Urol. 1998;159: 17–23.
13. Santa-Cruz RW, Leveillee RJ, Kongard A. Ex vivo comparison of four lithotripters commonly used in the ureter: what does it take to perforate? J Endourol. 1998;12:417–22.
14. Borboroglu PG, Amling CL, Schenkman NS, et al. Ureteral stenting after ureteroscopy for distal ureteral calculi: a multi-institutional prospective randomized controlled study assessing pain, outcomes and complications. J Urol. 2001;166:1651–7.
15. Ibrahim HM, Al-Kandari AM, Shaaban HS, et al. Role of ureteral stenting after uncomplicated ureteroscopy for distal ureteral stones: a randomized, controlled trial. J Urol. 2008;180: 961–5.
16. Thomas R. Rigid ureteroscopy: pitfalls and remedies. Urology. 1988;32:328–34.
17. El-Nahas AR, El-Tabey NA, Eraky I, et al. Semirigid ureteroscopy for ureteral stones: a multivariate analysis of unfavorable results. J Urol. 2009;181:1158–62.
18. Pearle MS, Nadler R, Bercowsky E, et al. Prospective randomized trial comparing shock wave lithotripsy and ureteroscopy for management of distal ureteral calculi. J Urol. 2001;166: 1255–60.
19. Aghamir SK, Mohseni MG, Ardestani A. Treatment of ureteral calculi with ballistic lithotripsy. J Endourol. 2003;17:887–90.
20. Sozen S, Kupeli B, Tunc L, et al. Management of ureteral stones with pneumatic lithotripsy: report of 500 patients. J Endourol. 2003;17:721–4.
21. Wu CF, Chen CS, Lin WY, et al. Therapeutic options for proximal ureter stone: extracorporeal shock wave lithotripsy versus semirigid ureterorenoscope with holmium: Yttrium-aluminum-garnet laser lithotripsy. Urology. 2005;65:1075–9.
22. Lee YH, Tsai JY, Jiaan BP, et al. Prospective randomized trial comparing shock wave lithotripsy and ureteroscopic lithotripsy for management of large upper third ureteral stones. Urology. 2006;67:480–4.
23. Sofer M, Watterson JD, Wollin TA, et al. Holmium: YAG laser lithotripsy for upper urinary tract calculi in 598 patients. J Urol. 2002;167:31–4.
24. Lam JS, Greene TD, Gupta M. Treatment of proximal ureteral calculi: holmium: YAG laser ureterolithotripsy versus extracorporeal shock wave lithotripsy. J Urol. 2002;167:1972–6.

25. Castro EP, Osther PJS, Jinga V, et al. Differences in ureteroscopic stone treatment and outcomes for distal, mid-, proximal, or multiple ureteral locations: the clinical research office of the endourological society ureteroscopy global study. Eur Urol. 2014;66:102–9.
26. Schuster T, Hollenbeck B, Faerber G, et al. Complications of ureteroscopy: analysis of predictive factors. J Urol. 2001;166:538–40.
27. Mariappan P, Smith G, Bariol SV, et al. Stone and pelvic urine culture and sensitivity are better than bladder urine as predictors of urosepsis following percutaneous nephrolithotomy: a prospective clinical study. J Urol. 2005;173:1610–4.
28. Chiu P, Chan C, Ma W, et al. Subcapsular hematoma after ureteroscopy and laser lithotripsy. J Endourol. 2013;27:1115–9.
29. Johnson B, Pearle M. Complications of ureteroscopy. Urol Clin N Am. 2004;31:157–71.

Chapter 8
Flexible Ureteroscopy: Available Instrumentation, How to Easily Traverse the Ureter, Procedural Risks and Potential Complications

Jonathan Cloutier and Olivier Traxer

Introduction

Stone disease remains a prevalent problem and an important aspect in the urologist's practice [1, 2]. Flexible ureterorenoscopy (F-URS) is gaining popularity and accessibility over the last two decades for the treatment of ureteral and renal stones. The smaller diameter, durability and maneuverability of the ureteroscope continues to evolve and contribute to the increased effectiveness of this treatment. Studies demonstrating the feasibility and safety of F-URS even in stones larger than 2 cm illustrate the versatility of this technique and the importance of being comfortable with all the equipment available in order to perform a successful surgery [3–5]. F-URS is presently a treatment option for stones of all sizes and locations in the ureter. In this chapter, we review the instrumentation available, the methods to navigate the ureter and potential complications of F-URS. The specifics regarding ureteral stents, guidewires, baskets, laser lithotripsy and other devices are discussed in other chapters. As proximal ureteral stones can sometimes be relocated or moved into the renal pelvis via retropulsion, we will also touch upon the use of flexible ureteroscopy in the treatment of renal stones in this chapter as well.

J. Cloutier • O. Traxer (✉)
Department of Urology, Tenon Hospital,
Pierre et Marie Curie University,
Paris, France
e-mail: jonathan.cloutier.2@ulaval.ca; olivier.traxer@tnn.aphp.fr

S.R. Patel, S.Y. Nakada (eds.), *Ureteral Stone Management: A Practical Approach*, DOI 10.1007/978-3-319-08792-4_8

Instrumentation Available: Flexible Ureterorenoscopes

In 1983, Bagley et al. described the use of a flexible ureteroscope, with the ability to flex 160° in one direction and 90° in the opposite direction [6]. Since that time, the technological advancements of F-URS have progressed at a remarkable pace.

Older Generation Flexible Ureterorenoscopes

The older generation of ureteroscopes are 70 cm long with a disk-shaped distal extremity of 7.4 French (Fr). The external sheath grows progressively from the distal to the proximal handle part (7.4–9Fr). There is a single 3.6Fr working channel that might allow up to 3.2 F instrument, and two or three fiber optic bundles, one or two for the illumination, and one for images transmission towards the endoscopic unit. The field of view of most ureteroscopes is 90° and the angle of view is 0°. The single working channel may have one or two connector luer-locks depending on the model, which allow for irrigation and simultaneous instrument placement.

Older generation flexible ureteroscopes have an active deflection of 180° downward and upward. Passive deflection can be attempted when the ureteroscope is advanced further into the collecting system with a fully active deflection. Most of the time, this maneuver can allow the scope to reach a lower pole calyx or advance further into a long lower pole infundibulum.

Newer Generation Flexible Ureterorenoscopes

The new generation of flexible ureterorenoscopes include an active deflexion of 270°, and have the standard ureteroscope characteristics in regards to its length and working channel characteristics (Fig. 8.1). The optics of the scopes vary between designers and rely on the number and quality of the fiber optic bundles used for illumination and particularly for image transmission. Depending on the number of fiber optic bundles, a honeycomb effect on the screen can be seen. An increased number of bundles will decrease the honeycomb effect, however these smaller fiber optic bundles may break more easily.

In 2001, the DUR-8Elite by ACMI became the first new generation flexible ureteroscope that had two levers: primary down (180°), primary up (170°), and secondary down (130°). Following the DUR-8Elite, other manufacturers produced the newer generation ureteroscopes, though these scopes had a single lever (Table 8.1).

Currently, with the arrival of the Olympus URF-P6 ureteroscope, each ureteroscope manufacturer produces a flexible ureteroscope with at least 270° of deflection in both directions. Moreover, some of the latest models are categorized as a "semi-flexible ureterorenoscope" (Fig. 8.2). A "semi-flexible ureterorenoscope" has more strength in the ureteroscope shaft and facilitates the ureteral ascension as well as

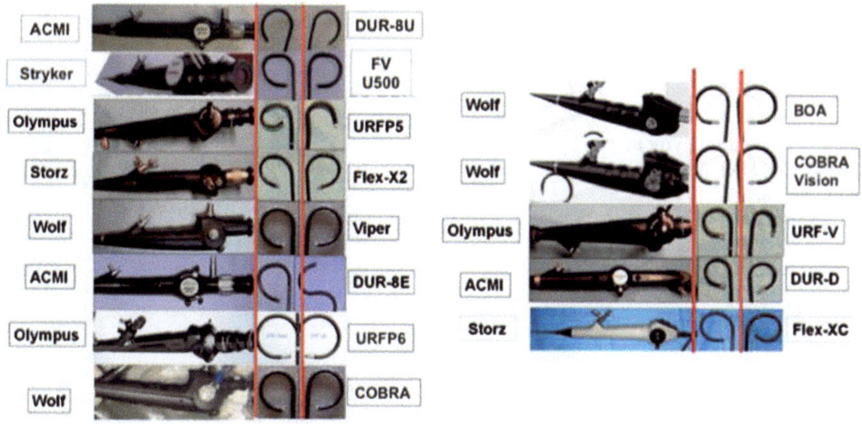

Fig. 8.1 Flexible ureterorenoscopes available. *Left* are fiber optic ureteroscopes, and on the *right* are the digital ureteroscope. The Olympus V2 is coming soon and is not illustrated

Table 8.1 Characteristics of different flexible ureterorenoscopes [7, 8]

Company	Product	Imaging system	Ventral deflexion (°)	Dorsal deflexion (°)	Tip diameter (F)	Shaft diameter (F)	Proximal diameter (F)	French scale test
Olympus Gyrus ACMI	DUR-8E	Optical	270	270	8.7	9.4	10.1	10
	DUR-8U	Optical	270	270	8.6	9.36	10.1	10
	DUR-D	Digital	250	250	8.7	9.3	10.1	11
Olympus	URF-P5	Optical	275	180	5.3	8.4	8.4	10
	URF-P6	Optical	275	275	4.9	7.95	7.95	10
	URF-V	Digital	275	180	8.4	10.9	10.9	12
	URF-V2	Digital	275	275	8.4	8.4	8.4	NA
Storz	Flex-*X*2	Optical	270	270	7.5	8.4	8.4	10
	Flex-XC	Digital	270	270	8.5	8.5	8.5	10
Wolf	Cobra[a]	Optical	270	270	6	9.9	10.3	11
	Viper	Optical	270	270	6	8.8	9	10
	Boa vision	Digital	270	270	6	8.9	8.9	NA
	Cobra Vision[a]	Digital	270	270	6	9.9	9.9	NA
Stryker	Flex vision U-500	Optical	275	275	6.9	7.1	7.2	10
Lumenis	PolyScope	Optical	180	0	9.6	8	8	10

E elite, *U* ultra, *NA* not available
[a]Dual channel

allows for increased scope control once in the renal pelvis during flexible nephroscopy. Other recent flexible ureteroscopes also tend to have a smaller tip with each scope fitting inside the 10/12F UAS [7] (Table 8.1).

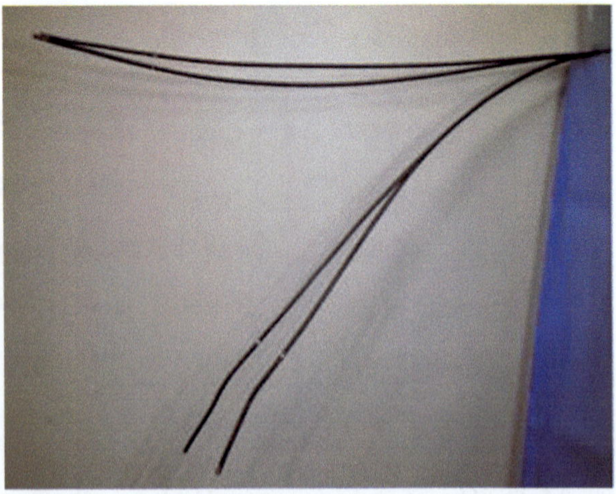

Fig. 8.2 The new ureteroscopes tend to be "semi-flexible." The newer Olympus URF-V2 and URF-P6 are at the *top* of the picture, and older Olympus URF-V and URF-P5 are both at the *bottom*

All current flexible ureteroscopes have acceptable optical quality with a 0° optic (except for a 9° optic for the Gyrus ACMI DUR-8Elite) and a field of view of 80–88°. The instruments are fragile and require manipulation and use with caution during the surgery as well as during the sterilization process. The surgeon should never insert an instrument into the working channel with a bent distal tip in order to prevent damage. With recent technological advances, the new generation of ureteroscopes are more durable and the utilization time before requiring a repair has increased up to 76 h longer compared to older generation of ureteroscopes. Some authors have also described performing up to 100 interventions with the same flexible ureterorenoscope without requiring repair [9, 10].

Newer Generation Digital Flexible Ureterorenoscopes

Since 2006, the digital optics technology has represented the next step in the development of endoscopy with a distal sensor. Studies have showed that the better image quality provides a higher precision for diagnosis, treatment, and a shorter procedure time (Fig. 8.3) [11].

The first ureteroscopes to use digital technology include was Gyrus-ACMI DUR-D Invisio, Karl Storz with the Flex-XC, the Olympus the URF-V and URF-V2, and the Richard Wolf Boa and Cobra Vision. These new ureteroscopes integrate a digital camera and light source in a single plug and play device. The principal disadvantages with the digital generation are that the distal tip diameter are slightly greater than the equivalent standard fiber optic ureteroscopes (Fig. 8.4). Nevertheless, the digital generation is now considered the gold standard in term of image quality.

All digital ureteroscopes by Karl Storz, Gyrus-ACMI and Richard Wolf use a Complementary Metal Oxide Semiconductor (CMOS) imaging sensor as a digital camera and a light-emitting diode (LED) as the light source. CMOS is a generic

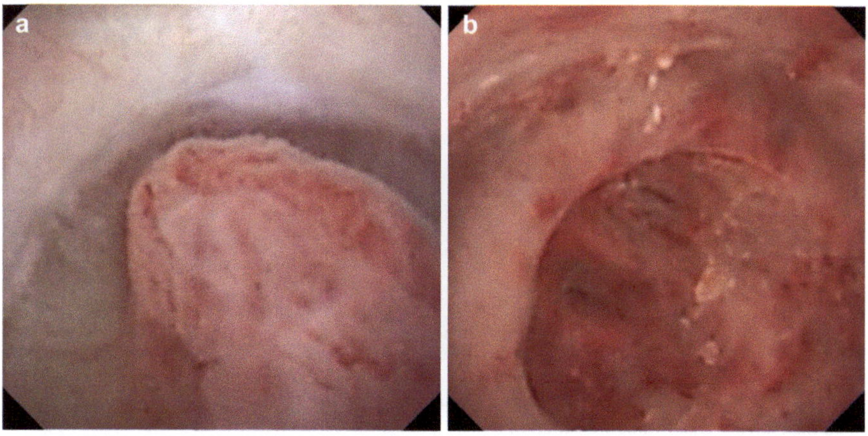

Fig. 8.3 Improved image quality of digital ureteroscopes: (**a**) Angioma of the renal papilla and (**b**) Papillary necrosis diagnosed in the context of hematuria

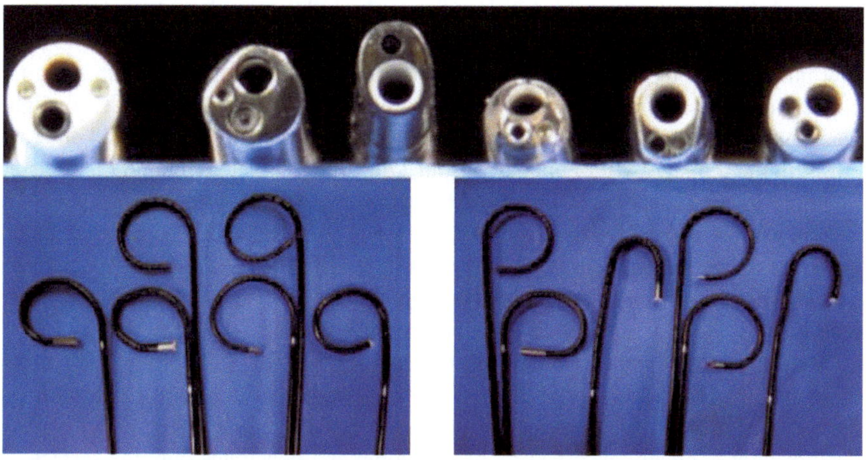

Fig. 8.4 Distal tips and active deflections for flexible ureteroscopes. *Left* is downward deflection and *right* is upward deflection. From *left* to *right*: Olympus URF-V, URF-V2, Storz Flex-XC, Olympus URF-P6, Storz Flex-*X*2, Olympus URF-P5

term for the process used to produce these image sensors, along with a multitude of other semiconductor items such as computer RAM processors like those from Intel and other manufacturers. CMOS image sensors can be made in the same fabrication as these other items, with the same equipment.

Olympus has introduced the URF-V incorporating a charge-coupled device sensor (CCD). Interline Transfer CCD consists of many Metal Oxide Semiconductor (MOS) capacitors arranged in a pattern that can capture and convert light photons into electrical charge, storing this charge before transferring it for processing by supporting chips. When recording color information, a color filter is placed over

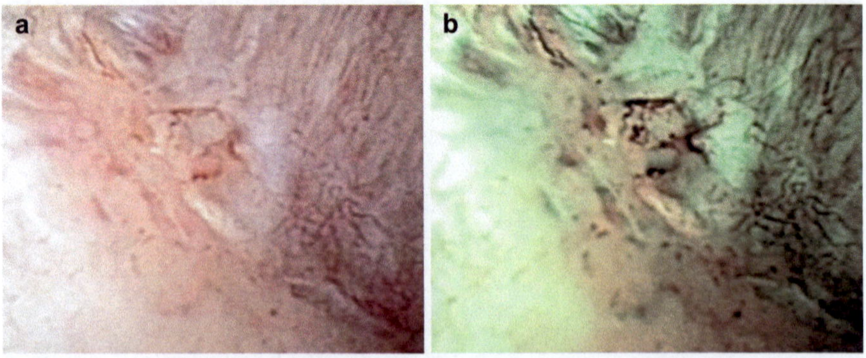

Fig. 8.5 (**a**) Upper tract urothelial tumor visualized with the white light. (**b**) Tumor visualized with the Narrow Band Imaging function

each light receptor making it sensitive to only one light color. This gives a value for one color at each pixel, and the surrounding pixels can provide eight more values, four each for the two remaining colors from which they may be interpolated from the original pixel. After the exposure is complete, the charge is transferred row by row into a read-out register, and from there to an output amplifier, analog/digital converters and on for processing. This row-by-row processing of the CCD's light data is where the sensor gets register and the rows behind it are each shifted one row closer to the register. After being "read-out," the charge is released, and the register is empty again for the next charge. CCDs rapidly attain high image quality but require a manufacturing process which is different from that used for manufacturing other computer chips such as processors and RAM. This means that specialized CCD fabrications have to be constructed, and they cannot be used for making other components, thereby making CCDs more expensive.

Moreover, the Olympus URF-V incorporates another new technology: the narrow band imaging (NBI) function. NBI is an optical image enhancement which narrows the bandwidth of the light production of the Olympus Exera II system. This narrow band of light is greatly absorbed by haemoglobin and penetrates only the surface of tissue increasing the visibility of capillaries and other delicate tissue surface structures by enhancing the contrast between the two. As a result, under NBI, capillaries on the surface are displayed in brown and veins in the sub-surface are displayed in cyan on the operating monitor. This technology is principally used in the detection or recurrence of urothelial tumors of the bladder or upper urinary tract. One of the current authors (OT) has demonstrated that NBI has the potential to improve the detection/recurrence of upper tract urothelial tumors by 22.7 % comparing to white light (Fig. 8.5) [12].

Disposable Flexible Ureteroscope

In 2009, the PolyScope by Lumenis became available. This is a disposable, modular flexible ureteroscope with a 70 cm working length and a distal tip size of 9.6F. It has a single-side active deflection of 180°, and the working channel is 3.6F [13]. Currently,

Fig. 8.6 Different guidewire tips

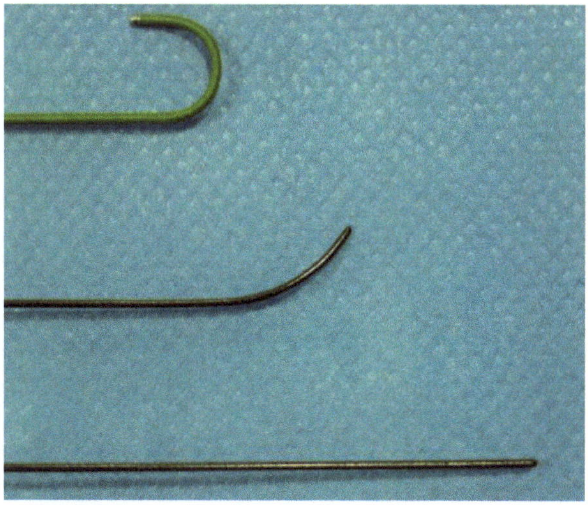

more studies are needed to demonstrate the efficiency and cost-effectiveness of this device though it does appear to be more difficult to manipulate than the usual flexible ureterorenoscopes.

How to Easily Traverse the Ureter

Getting ureteral access and reaching the proximal ureter or the renal pelvis can sometimes be challenging. Thus knowing alternative access methods to assist the endourologist is essential.

Ureteral Cannulation

Guidewires are well known to be essential during F-URS. Their use can be helpful for UAS placement or for the ureteroscope ascending a tortuous ureter and remain the best security during the surgery if a ureteral stent insertion is rapidly required. There are many types of guidewires and the description of guidewires is further discussed in Chap. 11. The authors strongly recommend using the stiff hydrophilic wires, where the first 3–5 cm are completely floppy hydrophilic to be less traumatic and the shaft of the wire is stiff and hydrophobic. Standard floppy tip polytetrafluoroethylene (PTFE) could also be used, but hydrophilic wire have been shown to be superior over the standard PTFE in gaining access to the renal pelvis when passing by a ureteral stone [14, 15]. The tip can be straight, angled or "J" tip and the surgeon, based on his/her own experience, will need to decide when he/she should use an angled one over a straight wire (Fig. 8.6).

When two wires are used and the flexible ureteroscope is placed over the working wire, you should use a hydrophilic wire to protect the working channel of the scope. Going up into the ureter directly over the wire facilitates the scope placement

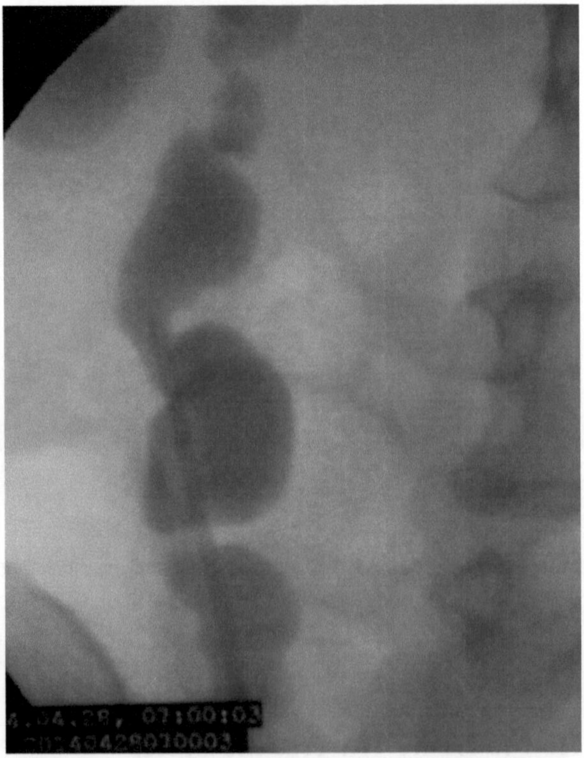

Fig. 8.7 Retrograde pyelography of a patient with an ileal ureter

into renal cavities. We strongly recommend using a safety wire even if the literature has demonstrated the feasibility of F-URS without a safety wire [16].

If difficulties are encountered in placing the guidewire during cystoscopy, a 5–7Fr open-end ureteral catheter can be used to accommodate the positioning of the guidewire into the ureter. The catheter is made of polyurethane and retrograde pyelography can also be performed in order to further delineate ureteral anatomy (Fig. 8.7).

Another use for the ureteral catheter is in the setting of a false passage caused during ureteral orifice cannulation. In this situation, a whistle tip ureteral catheter with a hydrophilic angled-tip guidewire can be used to help to find the correct passage into the distal ureter (Fig. 8.8). Following a right sided creation of a false passage, the correct way into the ureter is found by orienting the open-end and the angle-tip guidewire at 11 o'clock at the ureteral orifice. On the left side, you will have to orient the open ended catheter and angled guide wire to 2 o'clock.

Ureteral Access Sheath

The ureteral access sheath (UAS) was first developed in the 1970s to help gain ureteral access during ureteroscopy. One decade later, a peel-away sheath was introduced. The UAS has increased in use with the rapidly growing rate of retrograde intrarenal

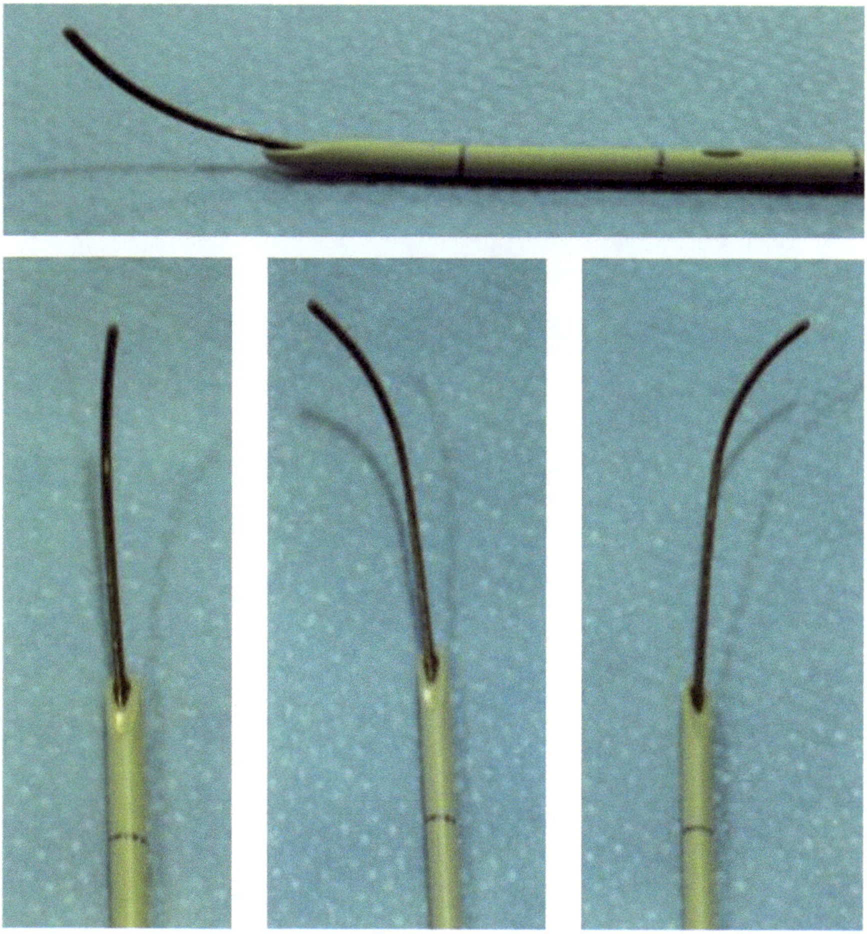

Fig. 8.8 Whistle tip ureteral catheter with angle-tip guidewire showed in different positions

surgery (RIRS) during the past few years. Using a UAS is not mandatory during RIRS, but it does allow easy repeat passage into and out of the ureter with the flexible ureteroscope. Moreover, it dilates the ureter and improves visualization by facilitating the return of irrigation. It also allows one to perform the surgery with lower intrarenal pressure thus reducing the risk of intrarenal reflux. It encourages the passage of small stone fragments and protects the flexible ureteroscope and gives more stability to the scope that permits optimal control during instrumentation into the renal pelvis [17].

The last generation of UAS has the unique characteristic of allowing the guidewire to exit on the side of the inner dilator just before the sheath (Fig. 8.9). Thus while removing the inner part of the UAS, the guidewire slides out on the side slit and thus becomes the safety wire (Fig. 8.10). This eliminates the need for multiple manipulations in order to place a second safety wire and allows one to remove the sheath in block with a stone when it does not pass into the UAS but pass only into the ureter. The UAS can be promptly replaced following its removal without the need for a second wire.

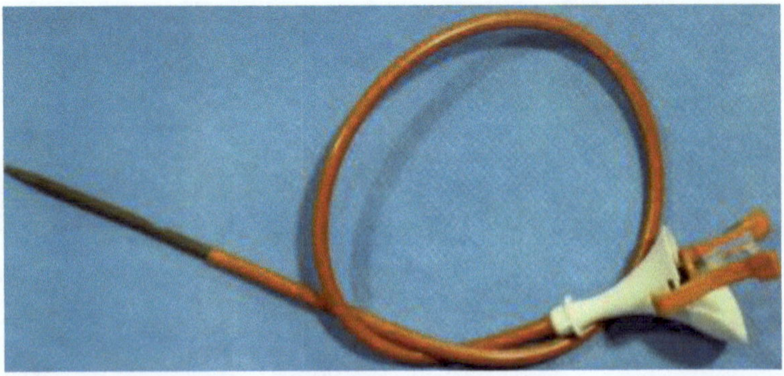

Fig. 8.9 Re-Trace by Colopast

Fig. 8.10 The guidewire slides out and becomes the safety wire

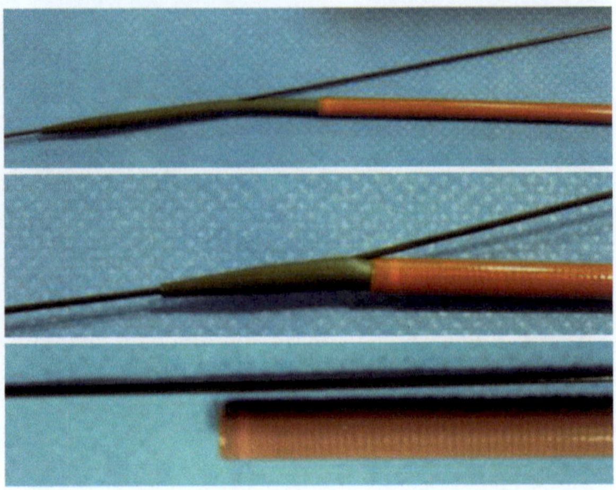

Since a normal ureter is 10Fr or less in diameter, we recommend using the smallest UAS possible in order to minimize ureteral trauma.

Irrigation Is Important

Constant basal irrigation with a manual hand pump is the authors' preference as it permits an increase in pressure only when required. The manual pump can be very useful during ureteral ascension as it helps to dilate the ureter, increases visibility and facilitates the navigation into the ureter (Fig. 8.11).

Details Regarding the Flexible Ureteroscope

Knowledge regarding different flexible ureterorenoscopes is important since diameter size and distal tip are different among the various scopes. Some

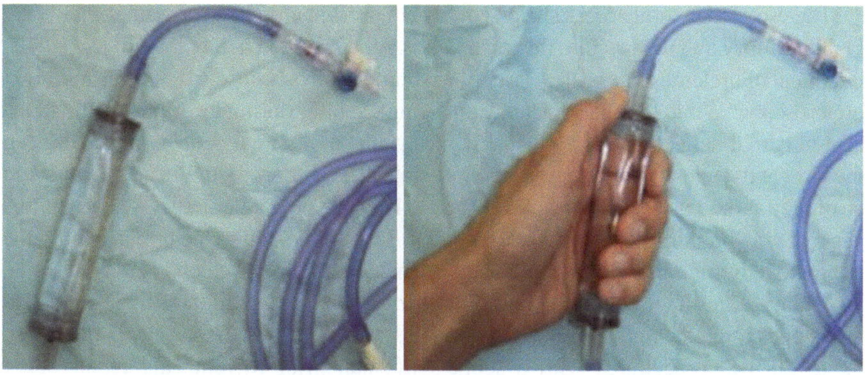

Fig. 8.11 Continuous irrigation with a manual pump to increase the irrigation while needed (TraxerFlow, Rocamed)

ureteroscopes do not fit in certain UAS [7]. In cases of a narrow ureter which does not allow placement of a UAS or surgeon's preference to not place a UAS during F-URS, knowing the distal tip size and shape of the ureteroscope may help to understand why it is more difficult to navigate access up the ureter with particular ureteroscopes (Fig. 8.4). Currently, while facing a narrow ureter, the authors prefer to work with either the Storz Flex XC, Flex X2, or Olympus URF P-6, URF V-2 in order to optimize our success to reach the proximal ureter or renal pelvis.

As discussed earlier in the chapter, some of the last ureteroscope models are "semi-flexible ureterorenoscopes" and facilitate ureteral ascension with their stronger and slightly stiffer shaft. Furthermore, new flexible ureteroscopes tend to have a smaller distal tip (<8.4F) that helps to pass through a smaller UAS and thus easily access the renal pelvis [7].

Procedural Risks and Potential Complications

This portion of the chapter will discuss the potential complications of F-URS. F-URS has an overall complication rate of 10.1 % with the majority of patients developing minor complications [3, 27]. The management of many of these complications is further discussed in Chap. 15.

Instrumentation Damage and Durability

A flexible ureteroscope is an instrument that needs to be handled with care. Unfortunately, ureteroscopes are fragile, and care must be taken during its use and in its sterilization to maximize its lifespan. Many components can compromise the durability of an ureteroscope, and when using these devices, a number of principles should be kept in mind.

The use of a ureteral access sheath could help prevent ureteroscope damage and may facilitate entry and reentry into the renal pelvis, however the UAS is seldom used in the treatment of ureteral stones [9]. A laser fiber should always be inserted through a straight ureteroscope. While feasible, abstain from using the laser during the time that the scope is at maximal deflection if possible. When working at maximal deflection, avoid using the laser at its high-power laser setting if possible. The authors recommend starting with an energy at 0.6 J and frequency of 6 Hz and to keep the power below 10 W. The authors suggest grasping the stone in a basket as soon as possible and repositioning it into the upper pole to minimize maximal deflection when treating renal calculi [18–20].

Many studies have found the durability for the latest generation of fiber optic ureteroscopes range from 5 to 18 procedures [19, 20]. Some authors have achieved from up to 50–100 procedures with a scope's lifespan prior to requiring repair being approximately 75 h of instrument time usage [9, 10]. The new digital ureteroscopes have supposed increased maneuverability and durability. Current studies have reported repair requirement for these scopes occurring after 20–22 procedures [18, 21].

False Passage and Ureteral Injuries

In the literature, false passages occur more frequently when a guidewire negotiates the site of an obstructing ureteral stone with the rate of creation of false passage being approximately 1–8.3 % [22, 23]. While treating renal calculi, a false passage into the ureter is rare, but this can occur when trying to cannulate the ureteral orifice.

A standard ureter has a transverse diameter of up to 9–10Fr [24]. Currently, most of the urologists are using a 12/14Fr ureteral access sheath for renal stones. The shear forces during UAS insertion and the decrease in ureteral blood flow with excessive distention are directly related to ureteral lesions during RIRS [25]. The ureteral wall injury classification is illustrated in Table 8.2. Ureteral access sheath injury can be found in 46.5 % of patients with high grade injury (Grade 2, 3 ,4) in 13 %. A ureteral stent should be left in place for 4–6 weeks when a high grade injury involving smooth muscle is found [26]. Complete ureteral avulsion during RIRS is a rare complication, but urologists have to continue to be conscious of this possible complication and should avoid being in a dangerous clinical situations (such as trying to extract an impacted stone) that could increase the risk of avulsion (<0.1 %) [27].

Table 8.2 Endoscopic classification of ureteral wall injury after RIRS using UAS [26]

Injury grade	Endoscopic findings
0	No lesion found or only mucosal petechia
1	Ureteral mucosal erosion without smooth muscle injury
2	Ureteral wall injury, including mucosa and smooth muscle, with adventitial preservation
3	Ureteral wall injury, including mucosa and smooth muscle, with adventitial perforation (periureteral fat seen)
4	Total ureteral avulsion

Bleeding

Intraoperative ureteral hemorrhage is a rare complication and would require postponing the surgical intervention followed by ureteral stent placement. Studies reported significant bleeding in 0.25–2.1 % of ureteroscopy stone cases [3, 27]. Generally, when the bleeding is not significant, the surgery can be completed. One can prevent this complication by avoiding to completely suck out the urine within the renal pelvis (depressurization and mucosa suction) and by avoiding direct lasering of the urothelial mucosa.

Urinary Tract Infection, Pyelonephritis and Sepsis

Urine culture is recommended prior to intervention and when there is a positive culture, appropriate antibiotic therapy should be administered and a negative culture obtained before considering ureteroscopy. In uncomplicated cases, it might be acceptable to perform a urinary dipstick with microscopy for pre-operative screening [28]. The AUA/EAU guidelines recommend antimicrobial prophylaxis prior to ureteroscopic intervention.

Nonobstructive pyelonephritis is the main postoperative complication and is reported in 0.7–8 % of cases. Fortunately, septic shock is described as a rare complication with a rate of 0.4 % and it is critically important that appropriate antibiotic therapy be initiated on time and to make sure that no ureteral obstructing is present [27].

Lower urinary tract infection (UTI) and bacteriuria is a common post-operative. The incidence of UTI and bacteriuria post-ureteroscopy is 1–4 % and in most cases can be effectively treated with oral antibiotics [28, 29].

Ureteral Stent Discomfort/Migration/Encrustation

A ureteral stent is placed to ensure upper urinary tract drainage commonly following ureteroscopy for ureteral stones. The primary indications for ureteral stenting include ureteral injury, large stone burden, ureteral stricture, post ureteroscopy in a solitary kidney, chronic kidney failure, a prolonged surgery time and ureteral dilation during the case. Studies have shown that routinely stenting the ureter at the end of an ureteroscopy is not obligatory for uncomplicated URS [28].

Patients with a ureteral stent in place do have significant morbidity and decreased quality of life during the duration of ureteral stenting. Al-Qahtani and coworkers have reported a 47 % discomfort rate secondary to the ureteral stent and the CROES URS Study Group reported a 0.9 % readmission rate related to stent discomfort [27, 28, 30].

Literature regarding stent migration have reported a rate of 1–4.2 % [31]. We need to consider this complication when a patient is readmitted from the emergency room with increased pain or bladder symptoms (Fig. 8.12).

Stent encrustation is another rare complication and is usually secondary to a patient lost to follow-up or in the case of severe hypercalciuria or in indwelling stents in pregnant women [32] (Fig. 8.13).

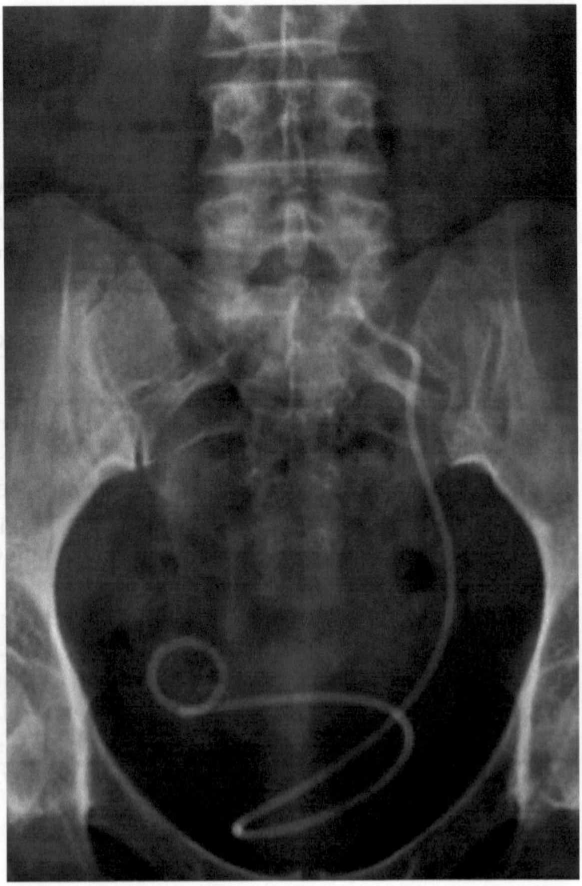

Fig. 8.12 Proximal loop migration of a ureteral stent

Pain and Renal Colic

Postoperative pain has not been very well documented in the literature. In some studies where ureteroscopy was used to treat stones larger than 2 cm have reported rate of 13–15 % for renal colic or pain following intervention. These complications were all considered minor, and were found to have resolved on their own (classified as Clavien Modified Classification Grade 1).

Steinstrasse

With the increased rate of F-URS and the utilization of ureteroscopy for stones larger than 2 cm, steinstrasse is a potential complication if all of the stone fragments have not been extracted. The literature currently reports a stenstrasse rate of 1.6–4 % with almost all patients requiring retrograde endoscopic intervention [3, 30].

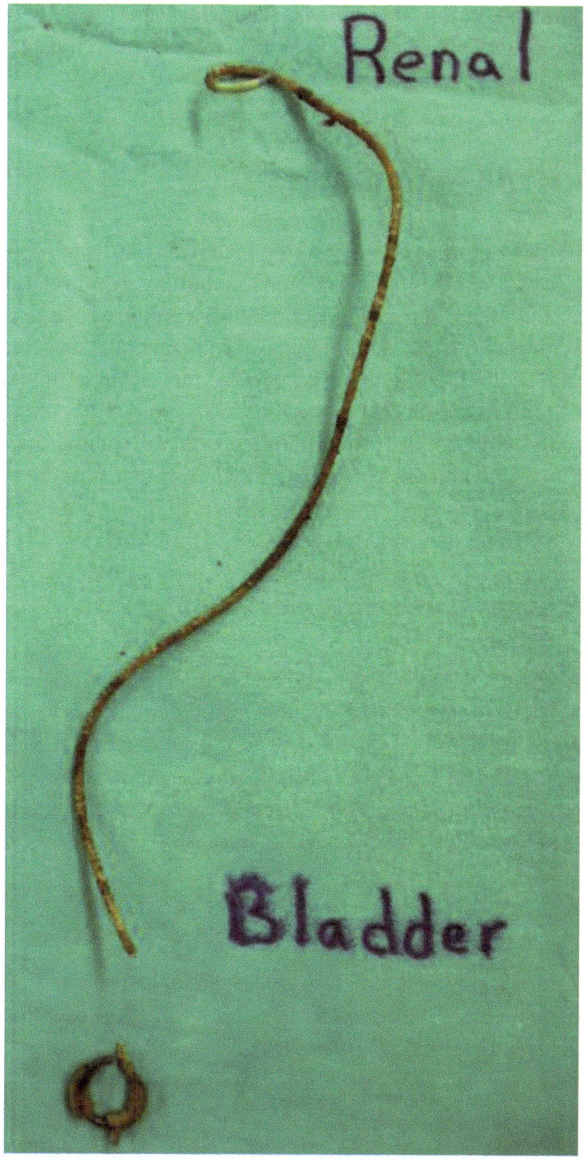

Fig. 8.13 Encrusted ureteral stent in a patient lost to follow-up following ureteroscopy

Hemorrhage and Transfusion

Intraoperative hematuria is a limiting factor to the completion of surgery due to limited visibility. Hematuria with a stent in place is to be expected as a common symptom of bladder irritation from the stent. Transfusion and clot retention are rare complications but have also been described [4, 27]. The rate of post-operative hematuria is relatively low with a range between 0.4 and 1.5 %, but patients with anticoagulation have maybe an higher rate [3, 27, 33]. The authors recommend informing the patient in the preoperative consultation that hematuria post-ureteroscopy may be common.

Ureteral Stenosis

Following ureteroscopy, ureteral stenosis has been reported from 0 to 4 % of cases. Ureteral stenosis can be related to intraoperative ureteral perforation, ureteral access sheath injury, too much friction with a ureteroscope or a previously impacted stone. With the current technological advancements, surgeon expertise and miniaturization of the flexible ureteroscope the rate of ureteral stenosis is fairly low (0–1 %). Careful insertion of a ureteral access sheath and manipulation of a flexible ureteroscope are necessary to minimize ureteral trauma and inflammation. Upper tract tumors treated via conservative management with repeated ureteroscopy may also have a higher rate of ureteral stenosis (9.3 %) [34].

Subcapsular Hematoma

In a review by Abourmarzouk and colleagues regarding renal stones treated by F-URS greater than 2 cm, subcapsular hematoma was seen in 0.8 % of treated renal units [3]. This complication represents 10 % of the overall complication rate which was 10.1 % (Fig. 8.14). Urologist needs to be aware of this potential complication particularly for a patient with long operative time and large renal stone burden.

Others

Additional complications in the treatment of stones via ureteroscopy that have been described are extrarenal stone migration (Fig. 8.15), acute urinary tract retention, acute prostatitis, cerebrovascular accident, pulmonary embolism and myocardial infarction [3, 29].

Complication Grades According to the Modified Clavien System

The authors recommend using the Clavien-Dindo classification for surgical complications in the reporting of complications of flexible ureteroscopy. This classification system has been shown to be reliable and is now recommended in both retrospective and prospective studies (Table 8.3) [35, 36].

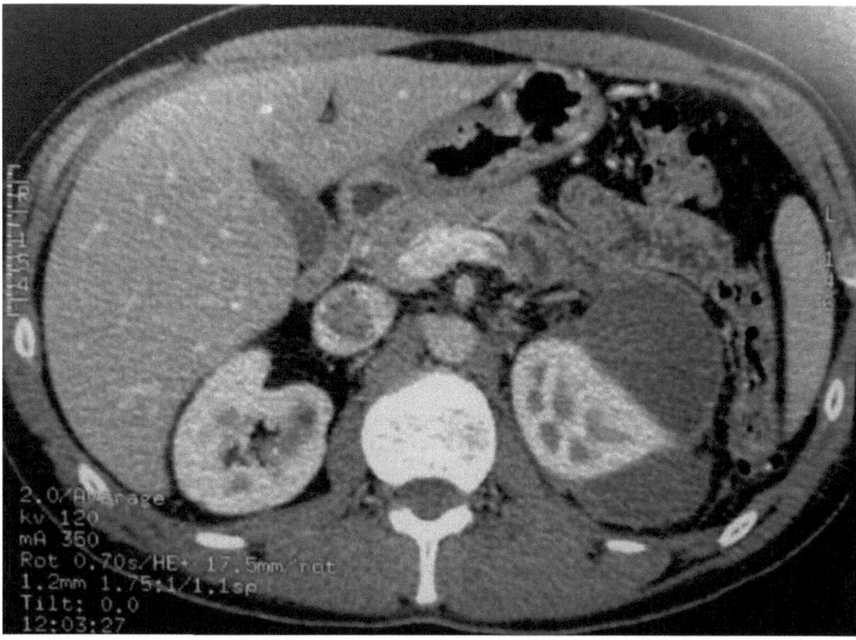

Fig. 8.14 Left subcapsular hematoma following F-URS for a stone larger than 2 cm

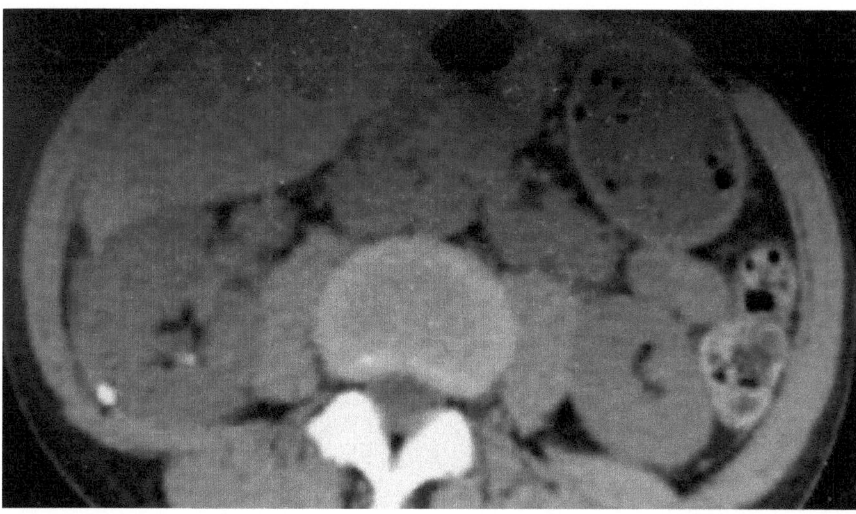

Fig. 8.15 During F-URS for a caliceal diverticular stone, the stone migrated outside of the renal cavities

Table 8.3 Classification of surgical complications [35]

Grades	Definition
Grade I	Any deviation from the normal postoperative course without the need for pharmacological treatment or surgical, endoscopic and radiological interventions
	Acceptable therapeutic regimens are: drugs as antiemetics, antipyretics, analgetics, diuretics and electrolytes and physiotherapy. This grade also includes wound infections plaies opened at the bedside
Grade II	Requiring pharmacological treatment with drugs other than such allowed for grade I complications. Blood transfusions and total parenteral nutrition are also included
Grade III	Requiring surgical, endoscopic or radiological intervention
Grade III-a	Intervention not under general anesthesia
Grade III-b	Intervention under general anesthesia
Grade IV	Life-Threatening complication (including CNS complications)[a] equiring IC/ICU-management
Grade IV-a	Single organ dysfunction (including dialysis)
Grade IV-b	Multi organ dysfunction
Grade V	Death of a patient
Suffix 'd'	If the patient suffers from a complication at the time of discharge, the suffix 'd' (for disability) is added to the respective grade of complication. This label indicates the need for a follow-up to fully evaluate the complication

IC intermediate care, *ICU* intensive care unit

[a]Brain hemorrhage, ischemic stroke, subarachnoidal bleeding, but excluding transient ischemic attacks (TIA)

Take Home Message

- F-URS is a viable treatment option for ureteral stones of all sizes and primarily in the location of ureteral stones in the mid/proximal ureter as well as renal calculi.
- Digital flexible ureterorenoscopes have improved durability and significant improvement in visibility which can further aid in stone treatment
- Obtaining ureteral access can be demanding and knowledge of the equipment and available instruments is necessary in order to assist the urologist during the procedure.
- In order to minimize complications during ureteral stone treatment, one must first be aware of potential complications during flexible ureteroscopy and when/why they may occur.

References

1. Stamatelou KK, Francis ME, Jones CA, Nyberg LM, Curhan GC. Time trends in reported prevalence of kidney stones in the United States: 1976-1994. Kidney Int. 2003;63:1817–23.
2. Scales Jr CD, Smith AC, Hanley JM, Saigal CS. Urologic diseases in America project. Prevalence of kidney stones in the United States. Eur Urol. 2012;62:160–5.

3. Aboumarzouk OM, Monga M, Kata SG, Traxer O, Somani BK. Flexible ureteroscopy and laser lithotripsy for stones >2 cm: a systematic review and meta-analysis. J Endourol. 2012; 26(10):1257–63.
4. Cohen J, Cohen S, Grasso M. Ureteropyeloscopic treatment of large, complex intrarenal and proximal ureteral calculi. BJU Int. 2013;111(3 Pt B):E127–31.
5. Hyams ES, Munver R, Bird VG, Uberoi JU, Shah O. Flexible ureterorenoscopy and holmium laser lithotripsy for the management of renal stone burdens that measure 2-3 cm: a multi-institutional experience. J Endourol. 2010;24(10):1583–8.
6. Bagley DH, Huffman JL, Lyon ES. Combine rigid and flexible ureteropyeloscopy. J Urol. 1983;130:243.
7. Al-Qahtani SM, Letendre J, Thomas A, et al. Which ureteral access sheath is compatible with your flexible ureteroscope? J Endourol. 2014;28(3):286–90.
8. Traxer O, Lechevallier E, Saussine C. Flexible ureteroscopy with holmium laser: the tools. Prog Urol. 2008;18:917–28.
9. Traxer O, Dubosq F, Jamali K, et al. New-generation flexible ureterorenoscopes are more durable than previous ones. J Urol. 2006;68:276–81.
10. Dedifidio L, De Dominicis M, Di Gianfrancesco L, Fuchs G, Patel A. Improving flexible ureterorenoscope durability up to 100 procedures. J Endourol. 2012;26(10):1329–34.
11. Somani BK, Al-Gahtani SM, de Medina SD, Traxer O. Outcomes of flexible ureterorenoscopy and laser fragmentation for renal stones: comparison between digital and conventional ureteroscope. Urology. 2013;82(5):1017–9.
12. Traxer O, Geavlete B, de Medina SG, et al. Narrow-band imaging digital flexible ureteroscopy in detection of upper urinary tract transitional-cell carcinoma: initial experience. J Endourol. 2011;25(1):19–23.
13. Bader MJ, Gratzke C, Walther S, et al. The PolyScope: a modular design, semidisposable flexible ureterorenoscope system. J Endourol. 2010;24(7):1061–6.
14. Liguori G, Antoniolli F, Trombetta C, et al. Comparative experimental evaluation of guidewire use in urology. Urology. 2008;72(2):286–9.
15. Clayman M, Uribe CA, Eichel L, et al. Comparison of guide wires in urology. Which, when and why? J Urol. 2004;171(6 Pt 1):2146–50.
16. Dickstein RJ, Kreshover JE, Babayan RK, Wang DS. Is a safety wire necessary during routine flexible ureteroscopy? J Endourol. 2010;24(10):1589–92.
17. Vanlangendonck R, Landman J. Ureteral access strategies: pro-access sheath. Urol Clin North Am. 2004;31(1):71–81.
18. Karaolides T, Bach C, Kachrilas S, Goyal A, Masood J, Buchholz N. Improving the durability of digital flexible ureteroscopes urology. Urology. 2013;81(4):717–22.
19. Monga M, Best S, Venkatesh R, et al. Durability of flexible ureteroscopes: a randomized, prospective study. J Urol. 2006;176:137–41.
20. Knudsen B, Miyaoka R, Shah K, et al. Durability of the next- generation flexible fiberoptic ureteroscopes: a randomized prospective multi-institutional clinical trial. Urology. 2010;75:534–8.
21. Multescu R, Geavlete B, Georgescu D, et al. Conventional fiber-optic flexible ureteroscope versus fourth generation digital flexible ureteroscope: a critical comparison. J Endourol. 2010;24:17–21.
22. Mushtaque M, Gupta CL, Shah I, et al. Outcome of bilateral ureteroscopic retrieval of stones in a single session. Urol Ann. 2012;4(3):158–61.
23. Geavlete P, Georgescu D, Nitä G, et al. Complications of 2735 retrograde semirigid ureteroscopy procedures: a single-center experience. J Endourol. 2006;20(3):179–85.
24. Zelenko N, Coll D, Rosenfeld AT, Smith RC. Normal ureter size on unenhanced helical CT. AJR Am J Roentgenol. 2004;182(4):1039–41.
25. Lallas CD, Auge BK, Raj GV, et al. Laser doppler flowmetric determination of ureteral blood flow after ureteral access sheath placement. J Endourol. 2002;16:583.
26. Traxer O, Thomas A. Prospective evaluation and classification of ureteral wall injuries resulting from insertion of a ureteral access sheath during retrograde intrarenal surgery. J Urol. 2013;189(2):580–4.

27. De la Rosette J, Denstedt J, Geavlete P, et al. The clinical research office of the endourological society ureteroscopy global study: indications, complications, and outcomes in 11,885 patients. J Endourol. 2014;28(2):131–9.
28. Türk C, Knoll T, Petrik A, Sarica K, Straub M, Sietz C. Guidelines on urolithiasis. Eur Assoc Urol. 2014. http://www.uroweb.org/gls/pdf/22%20Urolithiasis_LR.pdf.
29. Peyronnet B, Bensalah K. Complications of flexible uretero-renoscopies: prevention is better than cure. Prog Urol. 2013;23:F124–8.
30. Al-Qahtani SM, Gil-Deiz-de-Medina S, Traxer O. Predictors of clinical outcomes of flexible ureterorenoscopy with holmium laser for renal stone greater than 2 cm. Adv Urol. 2012; 2012:543–7.
31. Lividas KE, Varkarakis IM, Skolarikos A, Karagiotis E, Alivizatos G, Sofras F, Deliveliotis C, Bissas A. Ureteroscopic removal of mildly migrated stents using local anesthesia only. J Urol. 2007;178(5):1998–2001.
32. Ahmad I, Pansota MS, Tariq M, Saleem MS, Tabassum SA, Hussain A. Comparison between double J ureteral stenting and percutaneous nephrostomy in obstructive uropathy. Pak J Med Sci. 2013;29(3):725–9.
33. Aboumarzouk OM, Somani BK, Monga M. Flexible ureteroscopy and holmium: YAG lithotripsy for stone disease in patients with bleeding diathesis: a systematic review of the literature. Int Braz J Urol. 2012;38(3):298–305.
34. Johnson DB, Pearle MS. Complications of ureteroscopy. Urol Clin N Am. 2004;31(1): 157–71.
35. Dindo D, Demartines N, Clavian PA. Classification of surgical complications: a new proposal with evaluation in a cohort of 6336 patients and results of a survey. Ann Surg. 2004; 240(2):205–13.
36. Clavien PA, Barkun J, de Oliveira ML, et al. The Clavien-Dindo classification of surgical complications: five-year experienc. Ann Surg. 2009;250(2):187–96.

Chapter 9
Percutaneous Nephrolithotomy and Antegrade Ureteroscopy

Marcelino E. Rivera and Amy E. Krambeck

Introduction

Retrograde ureteroscopy has become a mainstay in the treatment of ureteral and renal calculi. From 2000 to 2010 there was a 127 % increase in the number of ureteroscopic procedures performed in the United Kingdom and it is anticipated that a similar rise in the number of procedures will be present in the United States [1]. A recent multi-institutional study of ureteroscopy found that there was a very low overall complication rate of 3.5 % and a high postoperative stone-free rate ranging from 85 to 95 % [2, 3]. Thus, it is not surprising that ureteroscopy is gaining acceptance as the primary treatment modality for upper tract stone disease. However, there are certain circumstances when retrograde ureteroscopy is not successful, such as altered anatomy or very large stone size. In such circumstances alternate treatment options must be considered. Antegrade ureteroscopy (URS) performed through a percutaneous approach is often a useful treatment option for proximal and mid-ureteral calculi when retrograde URS is not possible. The following chapter will discuss a brief history of percutaneous ureteral stone surgery, modern uses of antegrade URS, indications for antegrade URS, a description of current technique, and a discussion of postoperative management.

History

One cannot discuss the current role of antegrade ureteroscopy (URS) without first discussing a brief history of upper tract urinary calculi and management. While Fernström and Johannson were not the first to remove a stone percutaneously, they

M.E. Rivera, MD • A.E. Krambeck, MD (✉)
Department of Urology, Mayo Clinic, Rochester, MN, USA
e-mail: krambeck.amy@mayo.edu

S.R. Patel, S.Y. Nakada (eds.), *Ureteral Stone Management: A Practical Approach*, DOI 10.1007/978-3-319-08792-4_9

did describe the initial technique for establishing a percutaneous site for stone removal in 1976 [4]. They described the slow progressive dilation of a percutaneous established tract from the kidney to the collecting system of the kidney, utilizing a Couvelaire catheter that was 0.5 mm larger in caliber. The catheter was upsized on a daily basis to enlarge the percutaneous tract and allow for eventual removal of the upper tract stone material. Following the work of Fernström and Johannson, percutaneous techniques utilizing rapid tract dilation were reported in the United States and involved the utilization of metal, flexible or balloon dilators to dilate the nephrostomy tract up to 30 French (Fr) [5–7]. In 1982, Rusnak and colleagues, describe the initial technique of rapid dilation to 30Fr and utilization of an access sheath [5]. Utilizing their own design of polyurethane dilators the authors employed an 8Fr catheter over a guide wire and dilated the tract to 30Fr. To decrease friction and improve rigidity of the dilator a Teflon™ sleeve was used that remained in place during stone extraction. The current technique for percutaneous nephrolithotomy has been improved to a point where there is a relatively low overall complication rate, Clavien grade III or higher in <5 %, and a high overall success rate with retreatment rates of approximately 15 % [8]. The introduction of the percutaneous access sheath and flexible nephroscope now allows for safe inspection of the entire collecting system including the proximal ureter, with little concern for excessive bleeding or fluid absorption.

Prior to flexible nephroscopy allowing visualization of difficult to access areas, percutaneous ureterolithotomy was described in case reports as a means to treat an impacted ureteral stone without requiring an open ureterolithotomy. Clayman and colleagues [9] discussed direct percutaneous ureterolithotomy of a patient with an impacted proximal ureteral stone creating a ureteral diverticulum preventing access by flexible nephroscopy. After obtaining percutaneous access and passing a safety wire into the ureter, an aortography needle was placed directly to the stone, the established tract was dilated to allow a 30Fr working sheath, and a direct vision ureterotome was utilized to perform the ureterotomy. A stent was left in place and removed at 6 weeks with excretory urography at that time demonstrating no extravasation. Due to the potential significant morbidity of the case it did not replace open ureterolithotomy and technological advancements soon made both techniques obsolete.

While percutaneous nephrolithotomy became regularly utilized for large renal stone and proximal ureteral stones, the first reported series of antegrade URS was described by Gumpinger and colleagues in 1985 for the management of proximal ureteral calculi which were neither amenable to extracorporeal shock wave lithotripsy nor able to be flushed into the renal pelvis for percutaneous removal [10]. Their approach utilized a lower pole access with a balloon catheter placed distally to the stone to prevent propulsion. The rigid nephroscope was then inserted and after identification of the UPJ, the axis of the kidney was tilted to allow for visualization down the ureter. The nephroscope was removed, the sheath left in place and an 11Fr rigid ureteroscope was inserted to perform ureteroscopy. Mean operative time in the 22 cases was 55 min and postoperative hospital stay was 4 days. Ureteral perforation occurred in one patient.

Soon after the initial attempt of rigid antegrade URS, flexible antegrade URS was performed by Bagley and Rittenberg utilizing a rudimentary flexible ureteroscope [11]. Flexible antegrade URS was used to identify fragments passed down the ureter during percutaneous nephrolithotomy in eight patients. Flexible antegrade URS identified one obstructing fragment in their cohort. No complications were reported. The early version of flexible ureteroscopes did not have a deflection mechanism or working port, requiring irrigant to be supplied via an ancillary catheter or irrigation sheath. As technological advancements were made with decreasing diameter, increased length, and improved deflection of fiberoptic ureteroscopes, retrograde URS became common place in urologic practice. Antegrade URS was then reserved for patients with proximal ureteral stricture disease, large impacted calculi, patients unable to be placed in lithotomy due to severe joint disease, and patients with urinary diversion and previous unsuccessful retrograde access [12].

Modern Use of Antegrade URS

Today retrograde URS has become the treatment of choice for the vast majority of small and moderately-sized distal and mid-ureteral stones (<1 cm) and yields stone-free rates >90 % in the uncomplicated stone former. Even so, antegrade URS does have utility in the modern urologist's practice and has been demonstrated to result in higher stone free rates when compared with its retrograde counterpart. Sun and colleagues performed a prospective randomized study comparing percutaneous antegrade URS with retrograde URS for large, impacted proximal ureteral calculi [13]. Patients were randomly assigned to retrograde or antegrade treatment and mean stone size was 14.6 and 14.7 mm respectively. Length of hospital stay, procedure length of time, and return to baseline activities was longer with the antegrade group. However, stone-free rates immediately post-procedure, determined by KUB and ultrasound or CT in cases of radiolucent stones, and at 1 month postoperative were significantly higher in the antegrade group (95.3 % v 79.5 % and 100 % v 86.4 %, P=0.026 and 0.027 respectively). Maheshwari and colleagues also compared antegrade with rigid retrograde ureteroscopy for large (>1.5 cm) impacted upper-ureteral calculi in a nonrandomized series of 43 patients, 23 of whom underwent antegrade URS [14]. Complete stone clearance was achieved in one session in all patients using the antegrade percutaneous approach, while one session retrograde ureteroscopy was successful in only 55 % of patients, due to either stone retropulsion or secondary lower caliceal stones as verified with KUB. The authors concluded that antegrade URS can be performed in lieu of rigid retrograde URS for large impacted proximal ureteral calculi, without sacrificing stone free rates.

In developing countries with limited resources to newer technology, antegrade URS serves as a very effective means at achieving complete stone clearance without the morbidity of open surgery or the use of laparoscopy. Goel and colleagues reviewed their contemporary series of 66 patients with impacted ureteral calculi who underwent percutaneous antegrade URS for stone removal [15]. Of the 66 patients, 45 were accessed via a superior calix with nine supracostal and 21 via a middle caliceal puncture. A 26Fr rigid nephroscope was used in all cases with flexible nephroscopy used for stones which migrated distally. Complete clearance was achieved in 98.5 % of cases and all procedures were completed in a single session with one tract. Mean operative time was 47 min and aside from two ureteral perforations managed with stenting there were no other complications. The authors concluded that percutaneous removal of impacted proximal ureteral calculi in developing countries affords similar clearance rates with equipment that is more readily available, less expensive, and less fragile than flexible ureteroscopes.

Another important utilization of antegrade URS is in the setting of urinary diversion (either continent or conduit) after cystectomy or genital defects. Structural complications defined as ureteral anastomotic stricture or conduit stricture and urolithiasis are some of the most common complications following cystectomy and urinary diversion occurring in 11.5 and 15.3 % of patients respectively in a large cystectomy registry study [16]. Due to anatomic alterations it is sometimes not possible to access the upper urinary tract in a retrograde fashion once urinary diversion has been performed. Stuurman and colleagues describe antegrade flexible URS in urinary diversion patients for both stone and stricture disease [17]. There were 21 antegrade URS procedures performed, 15 of which were for stone disease. In the description of the technique patients were placed in the modified supine position, except for those with orthotopic neobladder in which the modified Valdivia position was utilized. Mean stone size was 13.4 mm and the stone free rate was 82.3 %. There were four complications in their cohort, two resulting in urinary tract infections treated with antibiotics and hematuria in the other two, which resolved spontaneously. Antegrade URS, when utilized for the proper indication, results in excellent stone free rates when compared to its retrograde counterpart.

Indications

Percutaneous antegrade URS is an ideal procedure for patients with preexisting ureteral pathology in which retrograde access cannot be obtained. Ureteral stricture disease leading to upper tract obstruction, patients with preexisting nephrostomy tube and patients with urinary diversion (Figs. 9.1 and 9.2) and reconstruction are well suited for antegrade URS in the setting of symptomatic ureterolithiasis. A large (>1 cm) impacted proximal or mid ureteral calculi or ureterolithiasis in the presence of nephrolithiasis requiring percutaneous nephrolithotomy are both excellent clinical scenarios where percutaneous antegrade URS is useful in patients without anatomic alterations. A ureteral stone located at the level of an iliac artery calcification or aneurysm can also be challenging to treat in a retrograde fashion and may be better suited for an antegrade URS approach (Fig. 9.3).

Preoperatively patients are counseled in the outpatient setting regarding the risks of antegrade URS and the typical convalescence. If a new percutaneous tract is established, overnight observation is recommended to assess for any significant

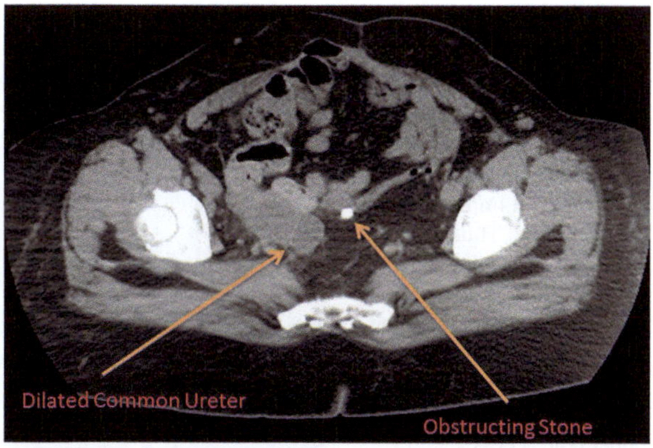

Fig. 9.1 Image of a female patient with an obstructing distal stone in the common ureter of her ureterosigmoidostomy. She was treated successfully with antegrade ureteroscopy

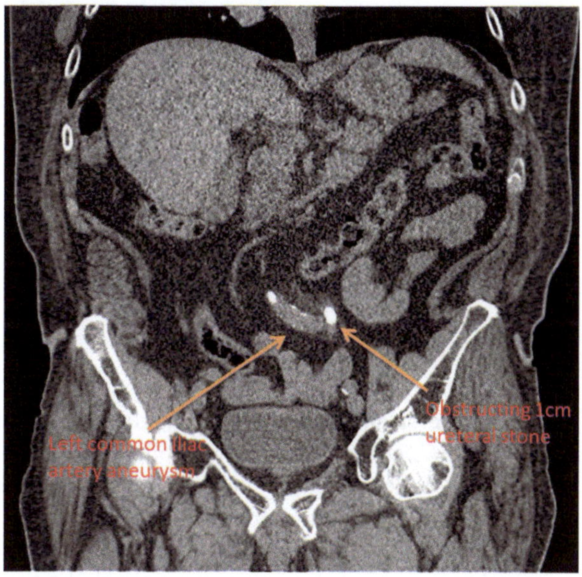

Fig. 9.2 Seventy-eight year old male with calcified common iliac artery aneurysm and 1 cm obstructing ureteral calculi

renal bleeding. If an established tract is utilized (i.e. patient already has indwelling nephrostomy tube), then the surgery may be performed as an outpatient procedure. All patients have a urinalysis with culture obtained as well as complete blood count and basic metabolic panel. All positive urine cultures should be treated prior to the procedure with culture-specific antibiotics. We recommend recent computed tomography (CT) imaging within the last 30 days to confirm stone size and location. Three dimensional CT imaging also provides information on surrounding organs and renal anatomy allowing for appropriate preoperative planning for the percutaneous renal access. If a new percutaneous tract into the kidney is created, a type and cross is obtained and patients are consented regarding the risk of blood transfusion.

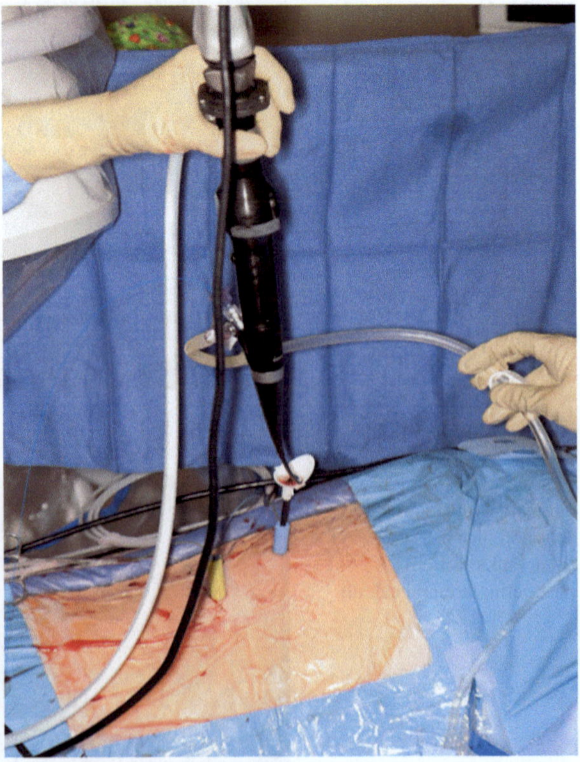

Fig. 9.3 Antergrade ureteroscopy performed with the two access sheath technique. This particular patient had a large lower and upper pole stone burden in addition to an impacted ureteral stone. Thus, two renal access sheaths are in place, one for the lower pole stones and one to access the upper pole and ureteral stone. A ureteral access sheath has been advanced through the upper pole access

Equipment

To perform percutaneous antegrade ureteroscopy the surgeon will require standard equipment for both percutaneous nephrolithotomy and for ureteroscopy. We recommend a rigid nephroscope, flexible nephroscope, and flexible ureteroscopy. Percutaneous access and establishing a percutaneous access tract using a renal access sheath should be performed as previously described [18]. Once a percutaneous renal access sheath is in place there should be a working wire in the ureter. A ureteral access sheath (13 or 14Fr outside diameter) can be placed through the 30Fr renal access sheath to the level of the ureteral stone. The ureteral access sheath facilitates stone removal from the ureter in an efficient manner (Fig. 9.3). A laser lithotripter, as well as stone basket for retrieval of fragments, is recommended. An ultrasonic suction device can also be helpful to remove stone debris or blood clots that collect in the renal pelvis at the time of the procedure. A ureteral stent and/or nephrostomy tube is used at the conclusion of the case.

Patient Positioning

We prefer placement of the patient in the prone position on a C-arm capable bed with careful attention paid to pad all pressure points. If we anticipate need for retrograde access to the ureter at time of antegrade ureteroscopy, then a prone split leg position is utilized. Stuurman and colleagues placed patients in both the modified supine position with elevation of the treated side and the modified Valdivia position, in which the patient is placed in a split leg position with the treated side raised as well in order to treat patients with urinary diversions [17].

Description of Technique

An understanding of renal and ureteral anatomy is vital when attempting antegrade ureteroscopy in particular when retrograde access has failed due to distal ureteral pathology. Our current practice utilizes triangulation technique for upper-pole percutaneous access as previously described [18]. Upper pole access is preferred as it allows for a direct course into the proximal ureter. Once access is established, a 0.038-in. hydrophilic nitinol glidewire is advanced down the ureter to the level of the stone. The wire is then exchanged for a stiff workable wire and the tract is then dilated using an 8/10Fr dilating catheter and a second stiff safety wire is placed through the 10Fr dilator. The working stiff wire is then used to advance the balloon dilator into the collecting system. The tract is balloon dilated and a 30Fr renal access sheath is then advanced into the kidney. Rigid nephroscopy is then performed to confirm appropriate sheath placement. An ultrasonic lithotripter with suction capabilities is often helpful to remove any blood clot or debris that may be present in the renal pelvis. Flexible nephroscopy is then performed to inspect the entire kidney and proximal ureter. If the flexible nephroscope cannot be easily advanced to the ureteral stone then a flexible ureteroscope will be necessary to complete stone removal. In order to facilitate easy access to and from the stone with the ureteroscope it is often beneficial to place a ureteral access sheath through the renal access sheath. Placement of the ureteral access sheath to the level of the stone is performed using a 12/14 or 11/13Fr sheath advanced with fluoroscopic guidance over the stiff working wire.

The ureteroscope is then easily advanced through the ureteral sheath to the stone. Once the stone is visualized laser lithotripsy is performed utilizing the holmium laser with settings appropriate for stone fragmentation (our preference is 8 Hz and 0.8 J). Stone fragments are then removed utilizing basket extraction. After all sizeable fragments have been removed, a guidewire is advanced down the length of the ureter and URS is performed for a full inspection of the ureter to the interior of the bladder. The ureteral access sheath is removed and the kidney is inspected one last time with the rigid and flexible nephroscope to remove any debris which may have migrated proximally. Next a double-J ureteral stent is deployed under fluoroscopic guidance. We generally leave the stent indwelling for 2–4 weeks depending on the degree of stone impaction and ureteral condition.

While our practice utilizes the "double sheath" technique for antegrade URS, a single ureteral access sheath-only technique can be utilized as well. Winter and colleagues describe a "no dilation" or "minimal dilation" approach with only the 12/14Fr access sheath passed antegrade over a guidewire which has already been passed down the ureter [19]. We prefer to have a renal access sheath in place to remove proximally displaced stones and concomitant renal stones which cannot be done with the single sheath technique.

If upper pole access cannot be obtained due to patient anatomy, a mid-pole or even lower pole access can be utilized. However, if the angle for the calyx to the ureter is too great then a ureteral access sheath cannot be used. In such cases, the ureteroscope is advanced down the ureter to the level of the stone visually. The stone material can then dusted it to very fine debris to be passed, with larger fragments extracted by basket. Such a technique can be very time consuming and tedious and is only recommended if all previously described options have been deemed inappropriate.

Postoperative Management

If upper pole access is established it is our practice to perform a postoperative chest x-ray to assess for any violation of the pleural cavity. Another acceptable option would be to fluoroscopically visualize the patient's lung fields prior to cessation of the surgical procedure. The patients are then monitored for 24 h and discharged postoperative day one. Antibiotics are continued for 1 week postoperatively or longer if stone culture is found to be positive for infection.

Follow-Up

A stone culture and analysis is performed on every patient. A positive stone culture is treated with culture-specific antibiotics. All patients are scheduled for follow-up 6 weeks post procedure with a 24-h urine supersaturation study and basic serum electrolyte studies including magnesium, phosphorus, calcium and uric acid. Imaging is performed based on American Urological Association recommendations and includes KUB and ultrasound for radiopaque stones or CT for radiolucent stones (i.e. uric acid) [20].

Conclusion

While retrograde ureteroscopy remains the standard treatment for many ureteral and renal stones, there are certain clinical scenarios when antegrade ureteroscopy is necessary. In appropriately selected patients the procedure can be performed in a safe and efficient manner resulting in excellent stone-free results and minimal morbidity. Utilization of both flexible and rigid instruments as well as various sized access sheaths can simplify the procedure and improve efficiency. A "double sheath" technique allows for removal of larger stone fragments and removal of renal stones during the same procedure.

Key Points

- While retrograde ureteroscopy remains the standard treatment for many ureteral and renal stones, there are certain clinical scenarios when antegrade ureteroscopy is necessary including ureteral stricture disease leading to upper tract obstruction, patients with urinary diversion and reconstruction, and large impacted proximal or mid ureteral calculi or ureterolithiasis in the presence of nephrolithiasis requiring percutaneous nephrolithotomy.
- Upper pole access is preferred to allow for placement of ureteral access sheath.
- A "double sheath" technique allows for removal of larger stone fragments and removal of renal stones during the same procedure.

References

1. Turney W, Reynard JM, Noble JG, et al. Trends in urological stone disease. BJU Int. 2012;109(7):1082–7.
2. de la Rosette J, Denstedt J, Geavlete P, et al. The clinical research office of the endourological society ureteroscopy global study: indications, complications, and outcomes in 11,885 patients. J Endourol. 2014;28(2):131–9.
3. Perez Castro E, Osther PJ, Jinga V, et al. Differences in ureteroscopic stone treatment and outcomes for distal, mid-, proximal, or multiple ureteral locations: The Clinical Research Office of the Endourological Society Ureteroscopy Global Study. Eur Urol. 2014;66(1):102–9.
4. Fernstrom I, Johansson B. Percutaneous pyelolithotomy. A new extraction technique. Scand J Urol Nephrol. 1976;10(3):257–9.
5. Rusnak B, Castaneda-Zuniga W, Kotula F, et al. An improved dilator system for percutaneous nephrostomies. Radiology. 1982;144(1):174.
6. Clayman RV, Castaneda-Zuniga WR, Hunter DW, et al. Rapid balloon dilatation of the nephrostomy track for nephrostolithotomy. Radiology. 1983;147(3):884–5.
7. Segura JW, Patterson DE, LeRoy AJ, et al. Percutaneous lithotripsy. J Urol. 1983;130(6):1051–4.
8. de la Rosette J, Assimos D, Desai M, et al. The Clinical Research Office of the Endourological Society Percutaneous Nephrolithotomy Global Study: indications, complications, and outcomes in 5803 patients. J Endourol. 2011;25(1):11–7.
9. Clayman RV, Preminger GM, Franklin JF, et al. Percutaneous ureterolithotomy. J Urol. 1985;133(4):671–3.
10. Gumpinger R, Miller K, Fuchs G, et al. Antegrade ureteroscopy for stone removal. Eur Urol. 1985;11(3):199–202.
11. Bagley DH, Rittenberg MH. Percutaneous antegrade flexible ureteroscopy. Urology. 1986;27(4):331–4.
12. Kim BS, Lee JN, Choi JY, et al. Antegrade flexible ureteroscopy for bilateral ureteral stones in a patient with severe hip joint ankylosis. Korean J Urol. 2010;51(11):800–2.
13. Sun X, Xia S, Lu J, et al. Treatment of large impacted proximal ureteral stones: randomized comparison of percutaneous antegrade ureterolithotripsy versus retrograde ureterolithotripsy. J Endourol. 2008;22(5):913–7.
14. Maheshwar PN, Oswal AT, Andankar M, et al. Is antegrade ureteroscopy better than retrograde ureteroscopy for impacted large upper ureteral calculi? J Endourol. 1999;13(6):441–4.
15. Goel R, Aron M, Kesarwani PK, et al. Percutaneous antegrade removal of impacted upper-ureteral calculi: still the treatment of choice in developing countries. J Endourol. 2005;19(1):54–7.

16. Shimk MS, Tollefson MK, Umbreit EC, et al. Long-term complications of conduit urinary diversion. J Urol. 2011;185(2):562–7.
17. Stuurman RE, Al-Qahtani SM, Cornu JN, et al. Antegrade percutaneous flexible endoscopic approach for the management of urinary diversion-associated complications. J Endourol. 2013;27(11):1330–4.
18. Miller NL, Matlaga BR, Lingeman JE. Techniques for fluoroscopic percutaneous renal access. J Urol. 2007;178(1):15–23.
19. Winter M, Lynch C, Appu S, et al. Surgery illustrated–focus on details: access sheath-aided percutaneous antegrade ureteroscopy; a novel approach to the ureter. BJU Int. 2011; 108(4):620–2.
20. Basiri A, Simforoosh N, Ziaee A, et al. Retrograde, antegrade, and laparoscopic approaches for the management of large, proximal ureteral stones: a randomized clinical trial. J Endourol. 2008;22(12):2677–80.

Chapter 10
Ureteral Stents

Ben H. Chew, Ryan F. Paterson, and Dirk Lange

Introduction

Ureteral stents are a common tool in urology and particularly for the treatment of ureteral stones. Ever since the introduction of the modern stent by Finney in 1978, stent designs have been similar but with various modifications [1]. Most stents are comprised of materials based on plastics such as polyurethane or ethylene vinyl acetate and various patented polymer mixes. Most stents are comprised of two pigtail curls to prevent the stent from migrating out of the renal pelvis and bladder. To date, there has not been any stent design or stent material that has proven to be more comfortable or superior to any other stent.

When to Stent

Stents provide drainage from the kidney to the bladder and keep the ureter open. The main reason to stent in the setting of acute presentation of a ureteral stone is for patients presenting with an obstructing ureteral stone and infection. This has shown to be equivalent in treating sepsis compared to insertion of a nephrostomy tube [2]. One study has identified a quicker time to defervescence in those treated with a nephrostomy tube but overall outcomes were fairly equivalent [2]. When looking at quality of

B.H. Chew, MD (✉) • R.F. Paterson, MD
Department of Urologic Sciences, University of British Columbia, Level 6 - 2775 Laurel St., Vancouver, BC V5Z 1M9, Canada
e-mail: ben.chew@ubc.ca; paterson@mail.ubc.ca

D. Lange, MD
Department of Urologic Sciences, University of British Columbia, 2660 Oak St., Vancouver, BC V6H 3C6, Canada
e-mail: Dirk.lange@ubc.ca

S.R. Patel, S.Y. Nakada (eds.), *Ureteral Stone Management: A Practical Approach*, DOI 10.1007/978-3-319-08792-4_10

life measures, it was fairly equivalent between the two groups, but stented patients had more voiding symptoms as would be expected [3]. Decompression of the infected system to allow drainage and antibiotic administration is highly recommended in this situation followed by delayed definitive treatment of the ureteral stone.

There is good evidence that ureteral stents are not necessary following successful uncomplicated ureteroscopy where there is complete stone fragmentation, no perforation or infection [4]. However, patients who did have ureteral stents had a slightly lower, albeit non-significant, rate of urologic complications following ureteroscopy [5]. Despite the vast literature supporting not stenting following ureteroscopy, there are still two large groups of surgeons who routinely stent and those who do not stent after uncomplicated ureteroscopy [6]. Stenting after use of a ureteral access sheath does decrease postoperative complications and emergency room visits [7, 8].

Stents can be placed in the acute setting to treat obstructing hydronephrosis and pain. While it is common to place a stent to temporize the patient until shockwave lithotripsy (SWL) can be performed, ureteral stents have been shown to hinder the passage of stone fragments following SWL [9, 10]. Therefore, placement of a ureteral stent prior to SWL does not improve the rate of stone passage nor does it significantly prevent the occurrence of steinstrasse. Stents should only be placed for reasons of infection, acute renal injury, and unrelenting pain. There is no evidence to place a stent prior to SWL to promote stone passage.

Methods of Stenting

The two main methods of inserting a ureteral stent involve placing a ureteral stent over a guidewire—either through a cystoscope or visually placing it using fluoroscopy only. There are slight modifications to these two techniques that will help in various situations. Below are two different techniques for ureteral stenting.

Stenting Through a Cystoscope

1. Fluoroscopy is typically required to ensure that the stent is placed properly.
2. Lightly diluted contrast can be placed into the kidney and renal pelvis to highlight that area and identify when the ureteral stent is in the correct position.
3. A guidewire must be in placed in the kidney and confirmed by fluoroscopy.
4. Examine the stent for markings to (a) ensure you are inserting the correct end if one end is tapered or if it is a dual durometer stent and one end is meant for the kidney and the other for the bladder and to (b) familiarize yourself with markings of where the distal bladder curl will occur so that you do not push the stent too far into the ureter.
5. Place the stent over the guidewire and insert it through the working channel of the rigid cystoscope. The stent should be directly visualized through the cystoscope as it inserts over the guidewire into the ureteral orifice. Ensure that you do

not insert the distal marker that delineates the bladder curl too far into the ureter. The proximal portion overlying the kidney should be visualized using fluoroscopy and as the stent enters the collecting system, the guidewire can be slowly withdrawn to allow the kidney portion to curl.

6. The guidewire can then be removed while holding the pusher with the stent in the correct position and the stent is visualized within the cystoscope. A good bladder curl should be ensured with direct visualization.

TIP: To ensure a good renal coil, leave the suture string on during placement (even if you intend to remove it later). Leaving the string on the stent will give you the ability to bring the stent backwards as well as forwards to ensure good positioning. Once the guidewire has been slightly removed as the stent enters the renal collecting system, if a proper renal coil is not seen on fluoroscopy, gently pull on the string of the stent to move it backwards into the proximal ureter. Once the stent is there and has straightened here, use the pusher to push it back into the renal pelvis (without the guidewire being in the proximal curl) and this will allow the curl to coil nicely. To remove the string, ensure you can see the stent in proper position either cystoscopically or fluoroscopically, cut the string loop and pull the string out *while holding the pusher to keep the stent in proper position*. This should be monitored cystoscopically or fluoroscopically.

Stenting Using Fluoroscopy

1. Lightly diluted contrast can be placed into the kidney and renal pelvis to highlight that area and identify when the ureteral stent is in the correct position. Be careful not to inject highly concentrated contrast as it makes the proximal curl of the stent difficult to visualize on fluoroscopy.
2. A guidewire should be in placed in the kidney and its position confirmed by fluoroscopy.
3. Insert the stent over the guidewire and use the pusher to advance the stent into the patient's ureter.
4. Maintain fluoroscopic surveillance of the bladder portion to ensure the stent does not coil up inside the bladder (which also leads to losing your guidewire access). Ensure the pusher end with the radiopaque marker is inserted first and look for this mark on fluoroscopy. A general rule of thumb is that this marker should be at the lower limit of the pubic symphysis for females and at the mid pubic symphysis for males to ensure that the stent is not inserted too far into the ureter. Be careful to adjust your landmarks in females with cystoceles: the limit is then much lower than the bottom portion of the pubic symphysis. These stents can almost be inserted just visually to the urethral meatus and then pushed into the bladder using a rigid cystoscope or Foley catheter given the short female urethra.
5. Once the stent pusher is inserted to the proper level, fluoroscopy of the kidney should be performed to ensure that the stent is in the renal pelvis. Slightly with-

draw the guidewire to allow the renal coil to curl in good position. If it does not coil properly, use the string to wiggle the stent backwards into the proximal ureter and then use the pusher again to push it into the kidney and it should curl nicely. (Remember not to hold the string while you are advancing the stent with the pusher, as these two opposing forces will not result in good stent positioning). If there is concern regarding the status of the proximal ureter (e.g. perforation), then care must be taken if the stent is pulled back into this area. If there is a known perforation, this technique should not be employed and the stent should not be pulled back into this area for fear that it may exit out the perforation.

6. Direct fluoroscopy over the bladder and observe that the stent pusher marker is in the correct position (mid symphysis for males, bottom of the symphysis for females) and then cut one end of the string (if you are going to remove it) and pull it out while holding the stent in place using the stent pusher. Continuous fluoroscopy should be used here to ensure the stent is not being pushed too far. Be sure to hold the end of the pull-string that contains the knot so that the whole suture can be removed smoothly through the stent hole. Remove the entire guidewire and the stent should curl nicely in the bladder.
7. If the bladder curl does not coil and is in the urethra, apply gentle suprapubic pressure which will often pull the stent into the bladder. Using the rigid cystoscope or a Foley catheter will also help move the bladder curl end of the stent into the correct position. If that fails, then direct visualization with cystoscopy is necessary to find the stent and push it or grasp it if needed and position the coil inside the bladder. Stents that are left across the bladder neck and sphincter will result in total urinary incontinence and are poorly tolerated requiring repositioning.

Problem: The Stent Is Too Short!

1. If the kidney coil is in good position, but the distal coil marker is well within the ureter (as seen through a cystoscope) or the stent pusher marker is above the desired location on fluoroscopy, the chosen stent length is too short. This is another reason to leave the string on the stent as it can simply be pulled back over the wire and exchanged for a longer stent. If a string is not present, the entire guidewire and stent can be pulled back as one unit to try and remove the stent. Cystoscopy and a grasper may be necessary to remove the stent. If this is done, remove the stent to the urethral meatus and pass another guidewire through it to preserve ureteral access.
2. To date, many measurements have been attempted to try and determine a surrogate marker that correlates well with ureteral length. These include height, torso length, CT length of the ureter [11–20]. The results appear to be mixed and the truest measurement is to use a ureteral catheter with graduated markings to directly measure the length of the ureter, although some of the other measurements (particularly CT) seem promising [12].

Problem: The Distal End of the Stent Is Pushed into the Ureter

1. If the stent is too short or a proper length stent is inserted too far into the ureter and nothing is visible within the bladder, this should be dealt with at the time of surgery rather than delaying repositioning. Such stents may not drain properly and may result in severe bladder symptoms from irritation of the ureterovesical junction. In some cases, it can result in severe hydronephrosis and if there is any ureteral or renal perforation, may lead to a urinoma.
2. Note: Leaving the string on the stent for positioning will often prevent this problem because if the stent is too short, it can simply be removed and exchanged for a proper length.
3. Rigid graspers with a semi-rigid ureteroscope can be used to remove the coil into the bladder to properly position the stent. Nitinol baskets can also be used, but can be tricky since the basket must be opened and placed *around* the <u>*end*</u> of the ureteral stent. This can be difficult since the space in the distal ureter is collapsed and not usually dilated. Furthermore, the nitinol basket can easily slip off the end of the stent when removing it from the ureter. If available, graspers offer the best method for grasping.

   An interesting technique that does not involve a ureteroscope is to place a guidewire into the ureter beside the misplaced stent. Insert a ureteral dilating balloon next to the stent and gently inflate (it does not need to be inflated to its nominal pressure), and then deflate the balloon. The deflated balloon forms folds and can create some friction and entrap the stent in the balloon and as the balloon is gently pulled back into the bladder, the misplaced stent can be pulled back with it [21]. If this is not possible, direct ureteroscopy becomes necessary to remove it. Care must be taken not to push the stent up the ureter even further using this technique. Insert the uninflated balloon under constant fluoroscopic guidance and stop if the end of the stent is being pushed up any further into the ureter. At that time, rigid ureteroscopy would be necessary.

Problem: The Stent Keeps Coiling in the Bladder

1. In some patients, particularly males with longer urethras and/or large prostate glands, there is simply not enough "purchase" to insert the stent properly and it continually coils in the bladder. If the coil becomes large enough, this can cause the guidewire and stent to come out of the ureter and for all of it to coil in the bladder, thus leading to loss of ureteral access.
2. This can be avoided by ensuring that there is proper **back-tension on the guidewire** while advancing the ureteral stent. In males, ensure the penis is put on stretch and straighten the guidewire in line with the penis as much as possible. Having the assistant hold guidewire taut and on slight back-tension (enough tension to make it taut without actually pulling it out) will help.

3. If the urethra is still too tortuous and the wire is coiling in the bladder, then switching to a stiffer guidewire may be helpful. In general, the softer the wire and the more hydrophilic it is, the more likely you are to lose access if there is any urethral tortuosity.
4. If the stiffer guidewire does not help advance the ureteral stent due to bladder coiling, "purchase" can be increased by removing the stent leaving just a stiffer guidewire and then inserting an 8F coaxial dilator over which a shorter 10F sheath is inserted. These are often obtained in dilation kits and the dilator and sheath come as a set. Insert the 8F dilator first followed by the sheath and then remove the 8F dilator. Be sure to insert the 10F dilator all the way to the urethral meatus in men to ensure that this sheath runs from the meatus directly into the ureter. This provides good backing for the stent as it runs though the urethra directly into the ureter. Therefore, the guidewire is no longer able to coil in the bladder. The stent is then inserted through the 10F sheath over the guidewire and the proximal portion is positioned using fluoroscopy as described above. The distal bladder curl is then positioned using fluoroscopy in the same manner, but before remove the guidewire, the 10F sheath must be removed while holding the pusher with the radiopaque marker visible under continuous fluoroscopy. Once the sheath has been pulled back, remove the string (if desired) and then the guidewire to coil the stent in the bladder. Pull-strings can still be left on if desired using this technique.
5. Another method with just a guidewire in the ureter is to backload the guidewire into the cystoscope and position the cope in line over the ureteral orifice. Rotate the beak of the scope that beak will prevent the guidewire from looping out medially within the bladder and then insert the stent through the cystoscope.

Problem: I Cannot Advance the Stent Past a Tightly Impacted Stone in the Ureter

If the intention is to insert a ureteral stent past an obstructing stone for delayed definitive therapy (e.g. shockwave lithotripsy, drainage of obstructive pyelonephritis, pain relief, etc.), this may pose a challenge in placing a stent through a tight area adjacent to the stone.

Obtaining guidewire access past the obstructing stone:

1. Ensure the guidewire is past the obstructing stone. If the guidewire does not go by the stone easily, remove the cystoscope and insert a 5 or 6F ureteral catheter to buttress the guidewire and try to gently probe past the stone. **TIP**: do not have the ureteral catheter directly adjacent to the stone, move it back about 5 mm so that the guidewire may be able to probe past the obstructing stone. The cystoscope often provides some needed resistance and backing to insert the guidewire; therefore, leaving the cystoscope in place may be helpful. Injecting dilute contrast through a ureteral catheter may also open up the plane between the impacted stone and the ureteral wall to try and dislodge the ureteral stone.

2. Change to a hydrophilic wire through the ureteral catheter and probe gently back and forth taking care not to perforate the area around the impacted stone which is often edematous and prone to perforation. Using an angled guidewire at this time may also be helpful as well. Inserting an angled angiographic catheter over the wire may also be helpful as well to bypass the impacted ureter.
3. If this is still not possible, insert an 8/10 Fr coaxial dilator and sheath leaving in just the 10 F sheath. This will help buttress the ureteral catheter. Again, try probing.
4. Exchange the ureteral catheter for an angled 5 or 6F angiographic catheter with the hydrophilic wire. Placing an angled hydrophilic wire provides two angled access points. When using an angled wire or catheter, be sure to probe and gently rotate the catheter and wire so that different combinations will provide different angles with which to attach the impacted stone. This double-angled combination of catheter and hydrophilic wire should be able to bypass all but the most impacted ureteral stones. Continue to rotate the angled ureteral catheter while probing and rotating the angled guidewire to attempt to pass the blockage.

   Inserting a stent past the obstructing stone:
5. Now that guidewire access is obtained, a ureteral catheter may be placed to (a) help dilate the area past the stone and to (b) inject dilute contrast to highlight the renal pelvis (this will help confirm the proximal coil being in the renal pelvis and to avoid unrecognized perforation of the guidewire and insertion of the proximal end of the stent outside the collecting system though a perforation).
6. If just a guidewire is present, a stent may be inserted over the wire making sure to provide good back-tension on the wire. If this does not provide enough purchase or buttressing to advance the stent, insert the 8/10F coaxial dilator and sheath leaving just the 10F sheath. Insert the stent through the middle of the 10F sheath which will give it more backing to buttress the stent past the stone.
7. Placing the stent over a super-stiff (±hydrophilic) wire through the 10F dilator may also be helpful.
8. If the above fails, the stone is too impacted and a decision must be made at this point to either place a ureteroscope (if available) and perform lithotripsy of the stone in order to make more room in the ureter to place a stent. In the setting of sepsis, more minimal lithotripsy is preferable and attempt to keep the amount of irrigation and pressure to a minimum to reduce the amount of intravasation of infected urine in the kidney. In the setting of obstructive sepsis, it is preferable to laser or treat the stone enough so that the stent can be placed. It is often tempting to completely treat the entire stone, but his can be dangerous and lead to even more overwhelming sepsis. If there is no sign of sepsis, more immediate treatment of the stone would be warranted such as more immediate shockwave lithotripsy or definitive ureteroscopy and lithotripsy.
9. Another option would be to stop the endoscopic procedure and perform a percutaneous nephrostomy tube either in the operating theatre or in the interventional radiology suite depending on the skillset and facilities available.

Problem: I Cannot Advance the Stent Past a Tight Area in the Ureter

If there is no obstructing stone in the ureter and a stent cannot be advanced past a tight area, the following may help:

1. Exchange your guidewire for a ureteral catheter and shoot a retrograde pyelogram to (a) highlight the anatomy of the area of narrowing and (b) to opacify the renal pelvis to confirm ureteral stent position.
2. If it is a stricture, serial or balloon dilators may be advanced to this area to open the stricture followed by stent insertion.
3. If there is no stricture, but only narrowing, then a 8/10Fr dilator and sheath can be inserted leaving only the 10Fr sheath. The guidewire is left through the 10F sheath and the stent can be advanced through the sheath. The 10F sheath will allow for more buttressing of the stent.
4. If still unsuccessful, a smaller caliber stent may be attempted. Many hospitals only carry one size of ureteral stent, but it would be prudent to have a small number of smaller diameter stents for such cases.
5. If the ureter is still to tight, serial dilators or balloon dilators may be advanced over this area to permit passage of a stent.
6. If nothing is successful and drainage is absolutely essential (e.g. perforation, acutely elevated creatinine from an obstructing stone that was successfully treated, or sepsis), then a 5 or 6 F ureteral catheter may be left in the renal pelvis for drainage and inserted into a foley catheter for drainage. The ureteral catheter will allow for passive dilation of the ureter and subsequent attempts at stenting can take place within a few days to a week or facilitate distention of the system with contrast for insertion of a percutaneous nephrostomy tube.

Post-operative Management

There is no evidence to support routine antibiotic use in stented patients following ureteroscopy and the AUA guidelines just recommend less than 24 h of antibiotics (pre-operative and peri-operative antibiotics) [22]. Stent symptoms are common including flank pain, dysuria, hematuria, infection and encrustation if left in long enough. To reduce the rate of stent symptoms, there is good Level I evidence to place patients on a daily alpha blocker until the stent is removed [23]. This is thought to relax the ureteral smooth muscle around the ureteral stent to reduce symptoms and improve patient tolerability.

There is no evidence on how long to leave ureteral stents after uncomplicated ureteroscopy, but the literature supports any time after 48 h to 7 days. Leaving a dangle string on the stent makes removal easier and does not have any disadvantages [24, 25]. There has been a case report, however, of a patient with a dangle string who removed only the string which broke and the stent was retained [26]. This example stresses how important patient education is in ureteral stenting.

Conclusion

Ureteral stents are often a necessary part of ureteral stone management. They can provide life-saving urine drainage in infected systems or facilitate drainage of the kidney after a ureteroscopic procedure. The decision on whether to stent following ureteroscopy that is uncomplicated (successful fragmentation of the stone, absence of infection and perforation) is the surgeon's decision as there is good evidence to support that they are not always necessary in these cases. There are several ways and tips on how to place ureteral stents for different scenarios. Insertion of stents for malignant ureteric obstruction is outside the realm of this book and can be reviewed elsewhere. Patient counseling is paramount prior to ureteral stent insertion to ensure they understand what symptoms to expect and that they understand they *must* have the stent removed at some point as it is only meant to be a temporary drainage device.

Take Home Points

- Ureteral stents are commonly used in urology today.
- There are different techniques on inserting a stent and various techniques when there is difficulty inserting a stent
- Maintaining a wide armamentarium of guidewires, catheters and stents is necessary to ensure patients will receive proper care.

References

1. Finney RP. Experience with new double J ureteral catheter stent. J Urol. 1978;120:678–81.
2. Pearle MS, Pierce HL, Miller GL, et al. Optimal method of urgent decompression of the collecting system for obstruction and infection due to ureteral calculi. J Urol. 1998;160:1260–4.
3. Joshi HB, Adams S, Obadeyi OO, Rao PN. Nephrostomy tube or 'JJ' ureteric stent in ureteric obstruction: assessment of patient perspectives using quality-of-life survey and utility analysis. Eur Urol. 2001;39:695–701.
4. Denstedt JD, Wollin TA, Sofer M, et al. A prospective randomized controlled trial comparing nonstented versus stented ureteroscopic lithotripsy. J Urol. 2001;165:1419–22.
5. Makarov DV, Trock BJ, Allaf ME, Matlaga BR. The effect of ureteral stent placement on post-ureteroscopy complications: a meta-analysis. Urology. 2008;71:796–800.
6. Auge BK, Sarvis JA, L'Esperance JO, Preminger GM. Practice patterns of ureteral stenting after routine ureteroscopic stone surgery: a survey of practicing urologists. J Endourol. 2007;21:1287–91.
7. Torricelli FC, De S, Hinck B, Noble M, Monga M. Flexible ureteroscopy with a ureteral access sheath: when to stent? Urology. 2014;83:278–81.
8. Rapoport D, Perks AE, Teichman JM. Ureteral access sheath use and stenting in ureteroscopy: effect on unplanned emergency room visits and cost. J Endourol. 2007;21:993–7.
9. Musa AA. Use of double-J stents prior to extracorporeal shock wave lithotripsy is not beneficial: results of a prospective randomized study. Int Urol Nephrol. 2008;40:19–22.
10. Mohayuddin N, Malik HA, Hussain M, et al. The outcome of extracorporeal shockwave lithotripsy for renal pelvic stone with and without JJ stent–a comparative study. JPMA J Pak Med Assoc. 2009;59:143–6.

11. Hruby GW, Ames CD, Yan Y, Monga M, Landman J. Correlation of ureteric length with anthropometric variables of surface body habitus. BJU Int. 2007;99:1119–22.
12. Shrewsberry AB, Al-Qassab U, Goodman M, et al. A +20% adjustment in the computed tomography measured ureteral length is an accurate predictor of true ureteral length before ureteral stent placement. J Endourol. 2013;27:1041–5.
13. Kawahara T, Ito H, Terao H, et al. Which is the best method to estimate the actual ureteral length in patients undergoing ureteral stent placement? Int J Urol. 2012;19:634–8.
14. Ho CH, Huang KH, Chen SC, Pu YS, Liu SP, Yu HJ. Choosing the ideal length of a double-pigtail ureteral stent according to body height: study based on a Chinese population. Urol Int. 2009;83:70–4.
15. Ho CH, Chen SC, Chung SD, et al. Determining the appropriate length of a double-pigtail ureteral stent by both stent configurations and related symptoms. J Endourol. 2008;22: 1427–31.
16. Jeon SS, Choi YS, Hong JH. Determination of ideal stent length for endourologic surgery. J Endourol. 2007;21:906–10.
17. Shah J, Kulkarni RP. Height does not predict ureteric length. Clin Radiol. 2005;60:812–4.
18. Paick SH, Park HK, Byun SS, Oh SJ, Kim HH. Direct ureteric length measurement from intravenous pyelography: does height represent ureteric length? Urol Res. 2005;33:199–202.
19. Norman RW, Breau RH. Optimal length of ureteric stents. Clin Radiol. 2003;58:257.
20. Pilcher JM, Patel U. Choosing the correct length of ureteric stent: a formula based on the patient's height compared with direct ureteric measurement. Clin Radiol. 2002;57:59–62.
21. Chin JL, Denstedt JD. Retrieval of proximally migrated ureteral stents. J Urol. 1992; 148:1205–6.
22. Wolf Jr JS, Bennett CJ, Dmochowski RR, et al. Best practice policy statement on urologic surgery antimicrobial prophylaxis. J Urol. 2008;179:1379–90.
23. Nazim SM, Ather MH. Alpha-blockers impact stent-related symptoms: a randomized, double-blind, placebo-controlled trial. J Endoruol. 2012;26:1237–41.
24. Barnes KT, Bing MT, Tracy CR. Do ureteric stent extraction strings affect stent-related quality of life or complications after ureteroscopy for urolithiasis: a prospective randomised control trial. BJU Int. 2014;113:605–9.
25. Bockholt NA, Wild TT, Gupta A, Tracy CR. Ureteric stent placement with extraction string: no strings attached? BJU Int. 2012;110:E1069–73.
26. van Diepen S, Grantmyre J. Broken retrieval string leads to failed self-removal of a double-J ureteral stent. Can J Urol. 2004;11:2139–40.

Chapter 11
Adjunctive Equipment for Ureteral Stone Management

Samuel Haywood and Sri Sivalingam

Introduction

The management of ureteral stones has evolved over the past several decades – where removal of ureteral calculi once required an open procedure, now virtually all calculi can be treated with a minimally invasive approach. This advancement has been fostered by significant technological improvements in both endoscopic visualization and dexterity. Instrumental in this transition has been the development and improvement of adjunctive tools used in ureteral stone management. The vast armamentarium available in endourology today not only requires the urologist to possess endourologic surgical skills, but also expertise and knowledge regarding the available equipment and proper use of each device. This chapter will provide an overview and discuss the practical application of the available ancillary equipment used in the management of ureteral stones.

Ureteroscopy

Ureteroscopy (URS) begins with obtaining access to the ureter, which in most cases, is achieved cystoscopically in a retrograde fashion; occasionally, however, access is obtained antegrade through an existing percutaneous nephrostomy tract. In either case, a guide wire is introduced into the ureter to enable access. A second wire may be introduced as a safety wire, although some experienced surgeons suggest this may not be necessary [1]. Once in position, the wires are used to introduce the ureteroscope into the ureter. The ureteroscope is then used to locate the offending calculus, wherein various working elements may be introduced to treat and/or remove the stone.

S. Haywood, MD • S. Sivalingam, MD (✉)
Department of Urology, The Cleveland Clinic, Cleveland, OH, USA
e-mail: HAYWOOS3@ccf.org; SRI.SIVALINGAM@GMAIL.COM

S.R. Patel, S.Y. Nakada (eds.), *Ureteral Stone Management: A Practical Approach*, DOI 10.1007/978-3-319-08792-4_11

Ureteroscopes

Paramount to successful outcomes in endourology is to select the most suitable ureteroscope for the task. Ureteroscope functionality depends on the size, visualization (optics and irrigation), and available working channels. Ureteroscopes can be categorized as semi-rigid or flexible, the former of which is basically a rigid scope that tolerates a small amount of bend. These generally provide better irrigation and visualization compared to the flexible ureteroscope [2]. However, the stiff shaft and narrow tip carries a potentially higher risk of damaging the urinary tract during insertion or use.

As opposed to the semi-rigid ureteroscope, the flexible ureteroscope has a flexible shaft that can be actively deflected to target the calculus. The flexible ureteroscope continues to improve with each generation, and this evolution includes decreased shaft diameter, improved deflection capability, and improved working channel calibers. The advantages of the flexible ureteroscope include improved maneuverability, longer length allowing access to all parts of the collecting system, and decreased risk of ureteral perforation. These advantages not only allow for superior performance with ureteral calculi in the upper third of the ureter but also allow for management of upper tract tumors or other pathology [2]. The main disadvantage of the flexible ureteroscope is the fragility of the device requiring the frequent repairs, and narrower/limited working channels. A full discussion of both semi-rigid and flexible ureteroscopes as well as the various models is provided elsewhere in the text.

Wires

The classic technique of URS begins with securing a guidewire into the upper urinary tract for obtaining and maintaining access during the case. Prior to the introduction of wires for endourologic application, access into the upper urinary system utilized ureteral catheters. The shift to the use of the guidewire represents a significant improvement, as the wire is thinner, better at bypassing obstruction, causes less trauma to the ureter, and can subsequently be used as a guide for introduction of additional equipment [3]. A large variety of commercially available wires can be used, which that vary across a number of characteristics – diameter, tip properties, shaft rigidity, and surface coating [4, 5]. The ideal guidewire would require little flexion force upon meeting resistance but a large force to puncture tissue [5]. The "margin of error" is the inherent difference between the ureteral perforating force and the force required to bend the tip [5]. That is, the wire that flexes too easily upon meeting resistance will also more readily slip out of position during manipulation, while a wire with a stiffer shaft will resist this tendency to slip but may require less force to perforate the ureter.

It should be stated that there is no unifying single ideal wire. A given procedure may require one to several different wires depending on the challenges encountered. Selection of the appropriate wire is instrumental in accessing and treating the ureteral stone while minimizing the risk of iatrogenic injury. For example, selecting a hydrophilic (i.e. slippery) guide wire may allow easy initial access to the difficult ureter, while switching to a wire with a stiffer shaft allows for increased stability for introducing other working elements.

Properties of Wires

The inner core of the guide wire is termed the mandrel and determines the rigidity of the wire [3, 6]. Common compositions of the mandrel are nitinol (a composite alloy of nickel and titanium) and stainless steel. The characteristics of nitinol give the metal a memory; i.e., it will return to its original shape after bending [7]. While this resists kinking, memory may allow movement of the wire after pressure is released resulting in change in wire position. Stainless steel wires have increased shaft rigidity compared to nitinol cores, but may kink permanently with various forces [3]. The use of this stiffer shaft may be used to straighten a tortuous ureter or as a guide over which to pass stents, sheaths, or other instruments. The Amplatz SuperStiff wire (Boston Scientific) is a commonly used stiff wire with greater shaft rigidity for passing additional tools. However, it is worth noting that attempts to backload a flexible ureteroscope over a stiff shaft wire can cause damage to the working channel of the scope [2]. To combat this risk, some manufacturers (e.g. Cook) have created SuperStiff wires with double floppy tips.

The outermost layer of a wire is an coating that decreases resistance during travel [2]. The two most common of these are the PTFE (polytetrafluoroethylene) or a hydrophilic coating. PTFE coating is considered the "standard" coating on wires and allows passage of the wire with low friction. However, certain situations (e.g. impacted calculus, tortuous ureter) dictate a need for a more slippery wire to pass the area of obstruction. As such, wires are used with hydrophilic coating which has a lower coefficient of friction to allow for easier passage. While hydrophilic coatings allow extremely low friction passage of the wire, wires with these coatings often do not have sufficient rigidity for passage of additional equipment, such as a ureteral stent, access sheath, or ureteral catheter. In addition, the slippery nature of these wires that makes them so beneficial for retrograde passage unfortunately is also responsible for a tendency to migrate or slip out of the upper urinary tract during manipulation [2]. In order to maximize the hydrophilic properties of these wires, they must be wet prior to use and kept moist during the procedure. If allowed to become dry, the coating may become "tacky" and difficult to use [3]. Examples of hydrophilic coated wires include the Glidewire™ (Boston Scientific) and NiCore™ (Bard Urological).

Other important properties of wires include the size and tip design. Wires range from 0.018 to 0.038 in. in diameter, with 0.035 in. and 0.038 in. sizes the most commonly used in adult ureters. Length of wires range from 145 to 280 cm [6]. The tips of wires often have different properties from the remainder of the wire, with the goal of presenting a safer leading edge. More specifically, the tips are designed to be

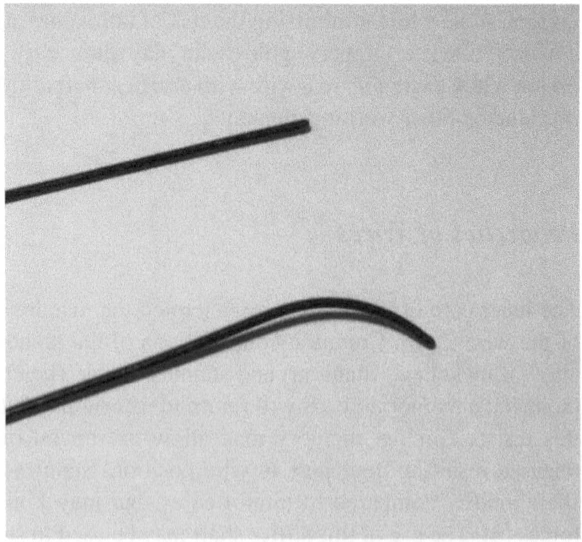

Fig. 11.1 Guidewires (*Straight tip* and *Angle Tip*, both Boston Scientific Glidewire)

flexible and soft in order to minimize ureteral trauma and allow maneuverability in the face of resistance [2]. The tip length can be variable, with the standard length being 3 cm. The Bentson-tip notably has a longer length of floppy tip (8–15 cm), which allows for extra curls of wire in the renal pelvis. This property makes a Bentson-tip wire especially useful as a safety wire [3]. The shape of the tip may be straight, angled, or J-shaped [3] (Fig. 11.1). The straight tip is the most common and is often the first choice in the setting of normal ureteral anatomy. The angle tip may prove useful in settings (e.g. prostatic hypertrophy with significant median lobe component) where the angle of approach to the ureteral orifice is unattainable with the straight tipped wire. The J-tipped wire is less common, but has a curl at the tip that presents an "elbow" at the leading edge that may reduce trauma to the ureter [3]. These may be useful in settings of impacted stone or significant ureteral edema. In addition, some wires as mentioned above are manufactured with dual tips on both the proximal and distal ends. The addition of a floppy tip to the proximal end of the wire allows for backloading the wire with decreased ureteroscope trauma [2].

More recently, hybrid guidewires have been introduced, which combine the beneficial properties of multiple types of wires (e.g. Sensor Wire™, Boston Scientific; UroWIRE XF™, Applied Medical; and U-Nite™, Bard Urological). In general, these wires possess a kink-resistant core, a distal tip with hydrophilic coating, and a soft proximal tip for backloading of a ureteroscope [2].

Comparisons of Wires

Given the variety available on the market, several groups have attempted to compare wire characteristics in order to help guide selection of the appropriate wire. Clayman et al. provided an early systematic comparison of guidewires, assessing two main functions - safe access to the upper tract and providing a guide over which to advance instruments [6]. The Boston Scientific Glidewire™ was suggested as the safest access wire, as it demonstrated the most lubricity and the safest tip. With respect to the ability to guide other instruments, the Amplatz super stiff guide wire demonstrated the greatest shaft rigidity. The rigidity of this wire was significantly greater ($p<0.05$) than all other wires tested.

In a comparison of hydrophilic wires only, Torricelli et al. compared wires with hydrophilic coatings on a variety of similar parameters [8]. Similar to the Clayman study, the Boston Scientific Glidewire™ was declared the safest wire to avoid perforations, secondary to the most flexible tip and highest force required to perforate a test sheet of aluminum foil. Notably, the Boston Scientific Zipwire™ had similar results with respect to tip perforation ($p=.340$ versus the Glidewire), but the higher shaft rigidity of the Glidewire ($p<0.001$ versus the other tested wires) suggested improved versatility for use with other instruments. It has been suggested that the very low coefficient of friction with hydrophilic coating may decrease tactile feedback and enable creation or propagation of a false passage.

Sarkissian et al. also provided a systematic evaluation of the hybrid guidewires [9]. Noteworthy is their comparison of shaft stiffness to the Amplatz SuperStiff and tip hydrophilicity relative to the NiCore™ and RadiFocus™ guidewire. They found that the Amplatz wire remained the stiffest wire available, with at least 34 % greater shaft bending force than the other wires, and accordingly, it continues to be the wire most suited to passing instruments. All in all, the wires produced by Boston Scientific (RadiFocus™, Sensor™, Amplatz) were noted to have lower tip bending force compared to the Bard-manufactured wires (U-Nite™, Ni-Core™), which confers greater applicability in the difficult ureter. Further, the RadiFocus™ wire showed the highest force required to puncture tin foil ($p<0.001$), and thus may be considered as one of the safest hybrid wires for initial access. Finally, it was noted that the Sensor™ wire had the highest coefficient of friction ($p<0.0002$), supporting its role as a safety wire with low risk of inadvertent migration.

While the above studies were performed in laboratory simulations, Liguori et al. tested several guidewires within cadaveric ureters [10]. As with other studies, the nitinol hydrophilic wires (Terumo Radifocus™, Boston Scientific Sensor™) were considered the safest for initial access. In fact, these two wires never perforated the cadaver ureter. Further, the Sensor™ had the lowest friction value of the tested wires, and was concluded to be the safest. Comparison was also made of several PTFE-coated wires, which would be considered more appropriate for passage of catheters or stents. Among those considered (Boston Scientific PTFE guidewire, Medtronic PTFE guidewire, and Emerald Cordis Guidewire), tip safety and friction tests were similar, but the superior resistance to bending of the Boston Scientific PTFE guidewire suggested it as the most preferable for use with introducing instrumentation.

Ureteral Dilation

After passage of guide wire(s), the ability to introduce further elements such as an ureteroscope, access sheath, or other instruments may be limited by a tight ureteral orifice, ureteral narrowing/stricture, or both. These may be related to normal anatomic variants, congenital abnormality, or related to prior medical treatment or surgery. The most common area requiring dilation is at the ureterovesical junction [2]. Ureteral dilation can be accomplished by coaxial dilators, ureteral access sheaths, balloon dilation, or interval ureteral stenting.

Coaxial dilation was the original method of ureteral dilation. This is accomplished by sequential passage of increasingly large dilators or a single tapered dilator. Both are passed over a guidewire to promote safe dilation. The use of a stiff shaft wire provides the best guide for passage of coaxial dilators. The main advantages of coaxial dilation include relative quickness of dilation as well as significantly lower cost compared to balloon dilation [11]. However, the dilation occurs via axial shearing force, which may cause mucosal injury and predispose the ureter to strictures [2, 11].

Ureteral access sheaths (UAS) can be considered a variant of coaxial dilation. These will be discussed in detail elsewhere in the chapter, but consist of an outer sheath with an inner tapered dilator. Together, these function similarly to a tapered dilator, but the inner portion is able to be removed, leaving the outer sheath for passage of ureteroscopes or other instruments. As the UAS is passed, the ureter is dilated similarly to with other coaxial dilators. This provides secure access proximal to the area of narrowing after dilation, but is again associated with axial shear forces that may damage the ureteral mucosa.

Conversely, balloon dilators provide radial dilation to the area of narrowing; force is exerted perpendicular to the mucosal axis, causing less mucosal damage [12]. The balloon catheters are between 4 and 7Fr in diameter, and balloon length can range between 2 and 10 cm [2, 3]. The system typically consists of a balloon situated around a central channel, which is used to advance the system over a wire. A second channel consists of tubing to the balloon for balloon inflation. The edges of the balloon length are marked with radiopaque markers ensuring knowledge of the outer limits of dilation with fluoroscopy. The important features to consider with any balloon dilators include the burst pressure as well as the compliance. The burst pressure of most ureteral balloons ranges between 8 and 20 atmospheres of pressure. The rupture of a balloon can cause significant damage to the urinary tract, so these products often package pressure gauges in the kit to ensure safe operation. The compliance of the balloon dilator determines its effectiveness, as a more compliant balloon may not overcome the deformity at the area of the narrowing, creating a classic hourglass appearance on fluoroscopy. The ideal balloon is therefore non-complaint, i.e., it will expand to 100 % of its designed diameter despite external forces. A comparison of ureteral balloons by Hendlin et al. assessed the balloon diameter and pressure with varying external compressive forces. This study demonstrated the Cook Ascend AQ™ balloon to be the most reliable balloon for use, as it reproducibly reached published diameter at the designated burst pressure. Notably, many balloons tested were not able to reach to target diameter even at burst pressure when subjected to larger external forces, which may limit the efficacy of these products [13].

Finally, the concept of interval ureteral stenting deserves mention. While not technically a dilation strategy, placing a ureteral stent during the acute stone episode to return at a later date for URS allows passive dilation. This is associated with significantly less chance of subsequent ureteral dilation. A study assessing predictive factors for balloon dilation during semi-rigid URS demonstrated fewer

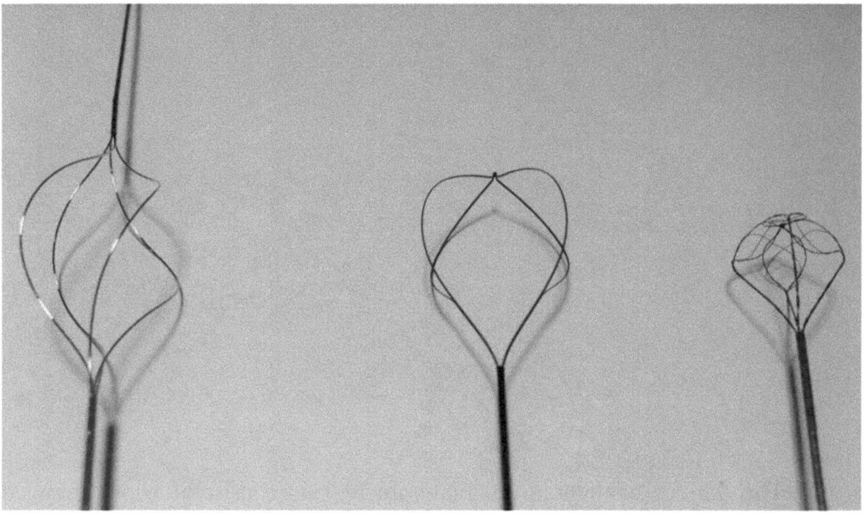

Fig. 11.2 Baskets examples: helical with tip (bard urological), flat (Boston Scientific), Multi-Wire (Cook)

requirements for dilation in patients with prior stent placement. Overall, dilation was performed in 27.5 % of procedures, while patients with prior stent required dilation only 1.8 % of the time [12]. In the setting of difficult ureteral access, this option may prove to be a safer strategy to avoid iatrogenic injury.

Manipulation Devices

Once the calculus is visualized, the ability to manipulate and/or remove it is dependent on the use of a manipulation device such as basket or forceps. Over time, the size of these devices has decreased enabling their passage through the working ports of most ureteroscopes. Baskets generally consist of several wires configured to surround the calculus to allow for manipulation, while forceps consist of two or more prongs that grasp the stone for manipulation. In general, both baskets and forceps rest within the shaft of the device, and are then extended beyond the shaft toward the target by the user using a handle at the end [14].

There are several characteristics of basket construction that must be considered for selection. As with guidewires, baskets may be composed of stainless steel or nitinol alloy [3]. The stainless steel baskets are stronger and may be preferred in a situation where ureteral distention is necessary for stone grasping. On the other hand, the elasticity of nitinol baskets may prove helpful in snaring eccentrically located stones. Further, the smaller size (in general) of nitinol devices allows for improved visualization through a similarly sized scope.

Another important characteristic is the wire configuration of the basket: flat-wire, helical, or multi-wire (Fig. 11.2). Baskets generally consist of 3–16 wires

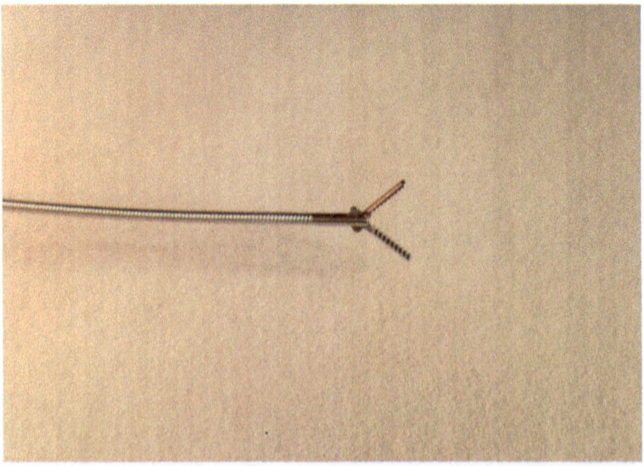

Fig. 11.3 Forceps example

arranged in various configurations. Flat-wire baskets consist of wires arranged concentrically. This is the most commonly used shape of basket. While it will reliably grab a target calculus, the shape may be less suited for manipulation of multiple calculi [3]. Helical baskets, as the name suggests, consist of wires that intertwine in a helical pattern around the target. This pattern grips the calculus securely, and as such may prove helpful for the entrapped stone, but the smaller openings may limit the size of calculus. Finally, multi-wire baskets consist of several wires arranged parallel to form a "canopy" [3]. This style may be most useful for removal of multiple calculi (Fig 11.3).

Some surgeons may choose use of a basket with a hollow core. This allows for passage of the basket over a wire or for advancing a laser fiber through the basket. The ability to pass a laser fiber may prove useful for performing lithotripsy on a stone held within the basket. Care must be taken to prevent striking the basket wires and potentially releasing a foreign body in the ureter.

Finally, the presence or absence of a tip is an important decision in basket selection. The tips extend beyond the cage of the basket, and in the ureter may help to negotiate a difficult ureter. However, a tip may prove to be dangerous, as it increases the risk for mucosal damage and/or perforation. As such, most baskets available today are of tipless design. If straightening a tortuous ureter is necessary with the use of tipless baskets, one can advance a guidewire first to assist with this.

Forceps consist of two or more prongs that extend from the shaft to grasp the target. They are different from baskets in that the prongs do not converge to a single point distally. Forceps may potentially be safer in the setting of larger calculi; i.e., if the stone becomes trapped in the ureter during removal, it may be more readily released, and reduce the risk of ureteral trauma or avulsion [3]. A comparison of various forceps and baskets in a porcine ureter model demonstrated that the simple two-prong forceps provided the fastest extraction for a single ureteral stone. The three-prong graspers were only slightly slower, but produced significantly higher tissue damage on macroscopic evaluation of the tissue. Within the baskets studied, the helical type basket provided the most efficient extraction in all models (single stone, impacted stone,

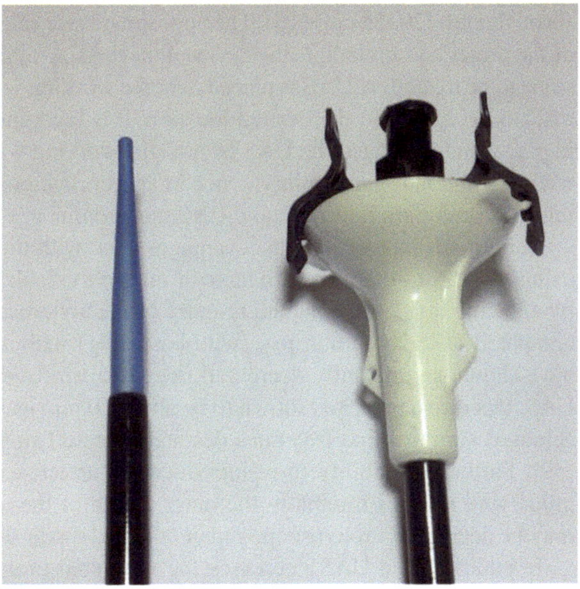

Fig. 11.4 Ureteral access sheath (cook)

steinstrasse) [15]. Comparison studies are available in the literature which evaluate individual basket types on applicable characteristics [16, 17]. While many baskets were tested, these studies found that the Sacred Heart Halo™ basket exhibited the best radial dilation, while the Cook N-Circle™ was the most expedient to extract a stone.

Ureteral Access Sheaths

The use of flexible ureteroscopes for calculus disease has drastically increased the abilities of the endourologist to treat ureteral calculi. However, difficulties still exist in their use. For example, it is common that complete removal of a ureteral stone may require several "passes" of the scope with a basket or forceps. This increases the chances of urethral or ureteral damage, and decreases the life of the ureteroscope as it is repeatedly passed over a wire. Further, the small irrigation channels of the flexible ureteroscope require significant pressure to allow adequate visualization. This pressure can transmit to the renal pelvis and cause increased pain or fluid absorption secondary to pyelovenous backflow. The ureteral access sheath (UAS) was introduced to address such concerns, and provide consistent, safe access to the ureter and kidney.

While various models exist, the basic design of the UAS remains the same (Fig. 11.4). A tapered dilator rests inside the outer sheath, connecting to provide a smooth, dilating surface. The outer sheath is usually coated with a hydrophilic coating to reduce the coefficient of friction and allow for smooth passage of the UAS. Options with the UAS include outer diameter (ranging from 9.5 to 16Fr) and sheath length (20–55 cm) [18]. The appropriate size selection depends on the caliber of the ureter and ureteral orifice, as well as the size of the ureter and location of the stone to be treated. A UAS is placed over the working wire and advanced under fluoroscopic guidance to the desired location. It is recommended to have a safety wire in place, and introduce the UAS over a stiff working wire to reduce the risk of wire buckling and iatrogenic injury. Once in appropriate position, the working wire and inner obturator are removed, and URS may commence.

Certain advantages and disadvantages exist with the use of the UAS. Certainly, using a UAS in situations with large or multiple calculi will decrease operative time by allowing quick removal and re-entry of the ureteroscope. Prospective trials have compared URS for lithotripsy (with basketing) with and without UAS, and these have shown significantly decreased operative time and cost in cases utilizing the UAS. Operative time was shown to be about 10 min less with the UAS in place, and achieved similar stone-free rates despite increased stone burden in the UAS group [19]. Further, the ability to re-introduce the ureteroscope without assistance of a guide wire reduces trauma to the inner sheath of the ureteroscope. As such, there may be decreased ureteroscope repair cost and repair downtime.

In addition, the UAS decreases the intrarenal pressure generated during URS by providing a pathway for irrigant outflow. The use of high-pressure irrigation systems during URS can be associated with very high intrarenal pressures. The specific effects of this short rise in pressures are not known, but theoretical concerns warrant minimizing pressures when possible. Further, it has been suggested that elevated intrarenal pressure increases pyelovenous backflow and subsequent fluid absorption [19]. Although prior studies have not shown significant fluid absorption, the theoretical risks may exist in patients with cardiac and/or renal dysfunction. One study utilized renal pressure measurements via percutaneous nephrostomy tubes during URS for ureteral calculi. It demonstrated decreased pressures in both the renal pelvis and parenchyma with the use of the UAS [20]. Further, the overall increase in flow of irrigation was associated with subjective improvement in visualization.

Concerns raised about the use of UAS centers on the effect on ureteral blood flow and associated stricture risk. While study of swine ureters has shown transient decrease in ureteral blood flow associated with UAS placement, compensatory mechanisms after removal demonstrated return of blood flow to near-normal levels. Further, histologic examination of these ureters did not demonstrate any evidence of ischemic damage to the ureteral wall mucosa [21]. Indeed, follow-up studies of patients undergoing URS with the UAS demonstrate similar rates of stricture to standard URS [2]. Regarding ureteral stent placement, un-stented patients post-URS treated with UAS were more likely to return to an ER post-operatively for evaluation (37 % versus 14 %) [18]. As such, it is recommended that ureteral stent be placed after URS if a UAS is used.

Much of the danger of UAS occurs during insertion of the sheath. The passage of the sheath into the ureteral orifice depends on both the coefficient of friction of the sheath and the axial force encountered by the UAS. If the axial force exceeds the buckling pressure, the UAS will buckle at the ureteral orifice and may cause damage to the urinary tract. Monga et al. tested eight different UAS with respect to buckling, kinking, and lubriciousness. The Cook Flexor™ sheath was suggested as the safest UAS to use, as this product had the highest buckling pressure (202 g of axial force) and was the most lubricious sheath tested [22]. The superiority of the Cook Flexor™ sheath was confirmed in a randomized trial of this sheath versus the Applied Access Forte™ sheath. No device failures were noted with the Cook sheath (compared to 44 % of cases with the Applied sheath) and subjective measurements by users also favored the Cook sheath (ease of placement, ease of instrument passage, ease of stone extraction) [23].

Irrigation Systems

Any successful endoscopic procedure requires fluid irrigation to allow adequate visualization. Irrigation systems may be passive, i.e., gravity based system with or without additional pressure, or actively through a provider-controlled mechanism. It is desirable to use only the least irrigation necessary in order to reduce stone migration and pressure effects on the kidney. Comparison of several irrigation systems showed that gravity-based systems provide less of an impulse to the stone [24]. However, the passive irrigation system may not provide enough irrigation pressure in more complex situations. Of the hand-held irrigation devices tested in these studies, the Boston Scientific Single-Action-Pump™ System was found to exert the least average maximum impulse on the stone, and also required the least frequent pumps to maintain a clear endoscopic field [24]. The Pathfinder Plus™ irrigation bulb (UTAH Medical) is another user-controlled irrigation device that allows for variable pressure delivery in a pulsatile or semi-continuous manner (Fig. 11.5).

Antiretropulsion Devices

The use of energy for stone fragmentation, regardless of type, can result in an impulse to the stone that can lead to retropulsion, i.e., retrograde travel of the calculus or fragments. Further, pressure from irrigation systems also adds to this tendency. This characteristic is undesirable as it may lead to increased operative time to retrieve these fragments or residual stone burden requiring additional procedures. Varying the type of energy may decrease retropulsion, but there are devices that aid in managing this tendency. Elashry et al. provide an extensive review of some of the available antiretropulsive devices [25].

Balloon based devices have an inflatable balloon mounted on a guidewire platform, allowing for efficient passage beyond the calculus. One disadvantage of this type of system includes the possibility of device rupture if contact is made with the lithotripter. Further, a significantly dilated proximal ureter may allow passage of fragments despite activation of the device.

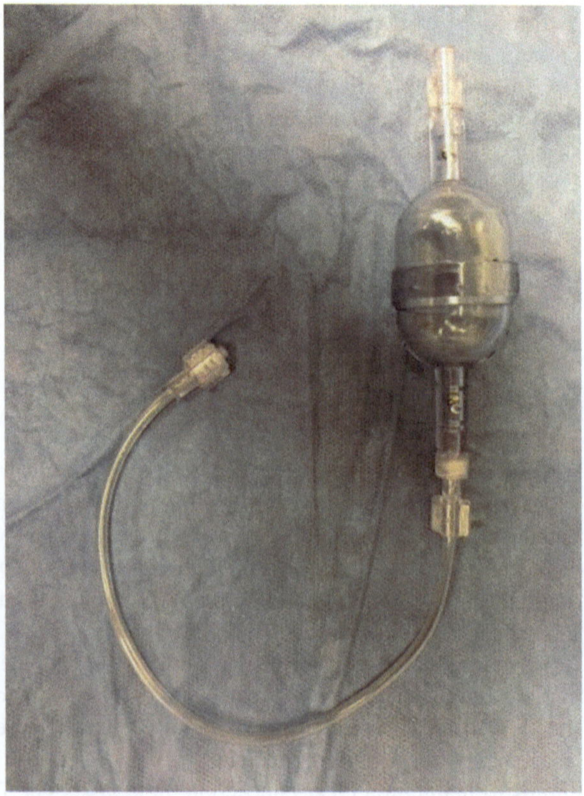

Fig. 11.5 Pathfinder Plus™ irrigation bulb (UTAH Medical)

A second type of antiretropulsion device is passed over a guidewire and provides a mechanical backstop to stone movement. In general, these are advanced over the wire proximal to the stone, the working element is deployed, and the working element forms a barrier. Examples of these include the Stone Cone™, PercSys Accordion™, or the Cook NTrap™ devices. All three have been shown in clinical trials to decrease stone migration [2]. The Stone Cone™ involves a PTFE sheath with concentric coils advanced over a nitinol wire that provides a backstop for stone retropulsion. The Accordion™ system consists of a deployable polyurethane film that prevents migration. Finally, the N-Trap™ basket involves a deployable backstop consisting of >20 nitinol wires forming a proximal barrier. Despite the varying design, all three have been tested in clinical trials demonstrating efficacy in preventing retropulsion [14]. A direct comparison of these three showed significant differences in performance characteristics (insertion/extraction force, radial dilation force, etc.), but all were noted to preventing proximal stone migration [26].

Chemical retropulsion devices have been developed recently. This involves the use of thermosensitive polymers that harden or liquefy depending on irrigant temperature [14]. These polymers are placed proximal to the stone, and the use of irrigation fluids result in hardening of the gel and formation of a backstop for stone migration. Once the stone is broken or manipulated, the use of colder irrigation

Table 11.1 Types of lithotripters

	Advantages	Disadvantages
Holmium laser	Low energy spread	High initial cost
	Effective against all types of stones	Limited life of fibers
	Smaller fragments, less retropulsion	
Electrohydraulic	Low initial cost	High risk of ureteral injury
	Can be used for several urologic issues	High risk of retropulsion → lower stone-free rates
Ultrasonic	Low risk to surrounding tissues	Only available as rigid probes
	Concominant suction abilities	
Pneumatic	Reusable probes	Rigid/semi-rigid probes only
	Energy source easily available	Significant retropulsion

liquefies the gel for removal of stone fragments [2]. Prospective trials of these polymers with respect to stone retrieval rates or remaining stone burden are not currently available, and further research is required.

Lithotripters

While the occasional calculus may be extracted simply by irrigation or gentle manipulation with basket/forceps, the majority of ureteral calculi are unable to pass primarily because the dimensions of the stone are too large for the given ureteral diameter. As such, performing lithotripsy to render calculi into fragments sufficiently small for passage or removal is an essential part of treatment of most ureteral calculi. Over the history of URS, several types of intracorporeal lithotripsy have been developed which merit discussion, although a more comprehensive discussion is provided elsewhere in this book. Advantages and disadvantages are summarized in Table 11.1.

Laser Lithotripsy

Laser energy has been used extensively in medical applications for many years, and its use in urology has greatly increased over the past few decades. Indeed, laser lithotripsy, and specifically Holmium: YAG laser lithotripsy, is the most common energy used in lithotripsy and can be considered the gold standard lithotrite with URS [2, 27]. Energy is transmitted from the laser fiber at a wavelength of 2,140 nm, which is highly absorbed by water [28]. Stone treatment occurs via photothermal ablation resulting in vaporization of the stone [2]. Because the energy is highly absorbed by water in the tissues, the thermal energy spread is only 0.5–1 mm, contributing to its safety profile [2]. Secondary to the limited energy spread, lithotripsy is performed by placing the laser fiber in direct or very close contact to the calculus. A laser fiber is composed of a fiber core, a cladding that surrounds the core, and an outer jacket [27]. Energy enters the core from the source at the proximal end, and is transmitted by internal reflection along the length of the fiber before being delivered to the target. Under normal circumstances, the light travels efficiently by total internal reflection. However, introducing bend to the fiber allows leak of the energy to the cladding/jacket, which may result in decreased efficiency or damage to the system [27].

Numerous types of laser fibers are now available. Fibers are often specific to the brand of generator used but can often be interchanged. The core of the fiber varies in size from 150 to 1,000 μm, although typically URS utilizes fibers at the smaller end of this range [27]. In addition, fibers are now produced with a ball-shaped tip at the distal end, which permits passage of the fiber through a deflected scope [27].

During operation of the system, both the pulse energy and pulse frequency can be varied. Notably, the use of higher pulse energy will more quickly provide fragmentation, but at the expense of larger fragments, greater retropulsion, and more rapid fiber degradation. Similarly, increasing pulse frequency allows more efficient energy delivery to the target, but the fast pulsations decreases the margin of safety if the ureteroscope moves within the ureter [27]. Most endourologists start performing lithotripsy at a known median setting (e.g. 0.6 J/6Hz, 0.8 J/8Hz) and adjust as needed during the case.

Compared to the other lithotripsy options, the Holmium laser provides several advantages. First, the short range of energy makes this a safe option with lower risk of ureteral mucosal damage. Second, the mechanism of action is effective against all types of stones [2]. Finally, the Holmium laser produces smaller residual fragments and less retropulsion of fragments than other lithotripsy energies [28]. This results in decreased operative time, operative cost, and risk of secondary procedures. Downsides of Holmium laser lithotripsy include the high initial cost of the energy source as well as the limited life of the fiber [27]. Of note, the Holmium laser generator also has other applications in urology (e.g. benign prostatic hyperplasia treatment and treatment of upper tract malignancies), which may help amortize the initial cost of the device.

Electrohydraulic Lithotripter (EHL)

In EHL, electrical energy is used to create a spark at the end of the probe. Once the probe is in direct contact with the stone, the spark causes vaporization of the surrounding liquid, followed by collapse of these cavitation bubbles that results in stone fragmentation [2, 29]. The EHL system is more commonly used in the treatment of bladder calculi. The appeal of the EHL system lies in the low initial cost and the ability to use the system in treatment of other urologic conditions. However, there is a significantly higher risk of ureteral injury, as the spread of energy is higher than in Holmium laser lithotripsy. In fact, early rates of ureteral perforation approached 40 % [2, 28]. In addition, there is more significant fragment retropulsion with the EHL, associated with lower stone-free rates [2].

Ultrasonic Lithotripsy

Ultrasonic lithotripsy is performed by high-frequency sound waves created by the generator, which are then transmitted directly to the probe. The vibration energy of the probe is then transferred into the stone, leading to resonance in the stone and subsequent fragmentation [30]. Ultrasonic lithotripsy is most common in percutaneous nephrolithotomy or cystolithalopaxy. The ultrasonic lithotripter proves to be beneficial for large stone burdens, where the superior efficacy is helpful. Another example of this is in the treatment of Steinstrasse following ESWL [29].

Ultrasonic energy is a safe form of energy, as surrounding tissue does not resonate and suffer damage [29]. Further, ultrasonic probes have the added benefit of concomitant suction through the hollow probe center to remove stone fragments, which increases efficiency relative to other forms of lithotripsy [28]. However, ultrasonic lithotrites are available only as rigid probes to allow transmission of sound energy, which limits their use in the ureter.

Ballistic/Pneumatic Lithotripsy

The pneumatic lithotripter works in a conceptually simple way. A rigid probe is placed in contact with the target calculus, and compressed air is used to accelerate an internal projective toward the stone. This energy is transferred to the stone, resulting in fragmentation [29]. An advantage of the pneumatic lithotrite is that the device may be reused and that the energy source (compressed air) is easily available [30]. As with ultrasonic lithotripsy, however, the mechanism of action requires a rigid or semi-rigid probe for effective fragmentation. Also, as one might expect from the type of energy, retropulsion of stone fragments is a significant problem [2].

Take-Home Points

- Hydrophilic wires provide safest ureteral access in settings of the difficult ureter.
- Use of a stiff guidewire provides a safe platform for introduction of working elements.
- Ureteral access sheaths can decrease operative time and increase stone-free rate for larger ureteral stones.
- Antiretropulsion devices demonstrate efficacy in reducing stone migration but have not yet gained widespread use among endourologists.
- Holmium laser remains the gold standard intracorporeal energy for ureteral stones given its applicability to all stone types and relative safety in the ureter.

References

1. Patel SR, McLaren ID, Nakada SY. The ureteroscope as a safety wire for ureteronephroscopy. J Endourol. 2012;26(4):351–4.
2. Duffey B, Monga M. Principles of endoscopy. In: Wein A, et al., editors. Campbell-Walsh urology. Philadelphia, PA: Elsevier Saunders; 2012. p. 192–203.
3. Rosenberg BH, Averch TD. Ancillary instrumentation for ureteroscopy. Urol Clin N Am. 2004;31(1):49–59.
4. Khanna R, Monga M. Instrumentation in endourology. Ther Adv Urol. 2011;3(3):119–26.
5. Holden T, Pedro RN, Hendlin K, et al. Evidence-based instrumentation for flexible ureteroscopy: a review. J Endourol. 2008;22(7):1423–6.
6. Clayman M, Uribe CA, Eichel L, et al. Comparison of guide wires in urology. Which, when and why? J Urol. 2004;171(6 Pt 1):2146–50.
7. Wainganker N, Okeke Z, Smith A. Guidewires and angled catheters. In: Monga M, editor. Ureteroscopy: indications, instrumentations and technique. New York: Springer Science+Business Media; 2013. p. 127–36.
8. Torricelli FC, De S, Sarkissian C, et al. Hydrophilic guidewires: evaluation and comparison of their properties and safety. Urology. 2013;82(5):1182–6.
9. Sarkissian C, Korman E, Hendlin K, et al. Systematic evaluation of hybrid guidewires: shaft stiffness, lubricity, and tip configuration. Urology. 2012;79(3):513–7.
10. Liguori G, Antoniolli F, Trombetta C, et al. Comparative experimental evaluation of guidewire use in urology. Urology. 2008;72(2):286–9; discussion 289–90.
11. Gaylis F, Bastuba M, Bidair M, et al. Ureteral dilation using a tapered dilator: a cost-effective approach. J Endourol. 2000;14(5):447–9.
12. Bin X, Friedlander JI, Chuang KW, et al. Predictive factors for intraoperative balloon dilation in semirigid ureteroscopic lithotripsy. J Endourol. 2012;26(8):988–91.
13. Hendlin K, Lund B, Dockendorf K, et al. Radial dilation of ureteral balloons: comparative in vitro analysis. J Endourol. 2005;19(5):575–8.
14. Foell K, Honey J, Pace K. Stone baskets and forceps. In: Monga M, editor. Ureteroscopy: indications, instrumentation, and technique. New York: Springer Science+Business Media; 2013. p. 179–97.
15. Ptashnyk T, Cueva-Martinez A, Michel MS, et al. Comparative investigations on the retrieval capabilities of various baskets and graspers in four ex vivo models. Eur Urol. 2002;41(4):406–10.
16. Korman E, Hendlin K, Monga M. Small-diameter nitinol stone baskets: radial dilation force and dynamics of opening. J Endourol. 2011;25(9):1537–40.
17. Lukasewycz S, et al. Comparison of tipless and helical baskets in an in vitro ureteral model. Urology. 2004;64(3):435–8; discussion 438.
18. Feia K, Duffey B, Anderson J. Ureteral access sheaths. In: Monga M, editor. Ureteroscopy: indications, instrumentation, and technique. New York: Springer Science+Business Media; 2013. p. 137–44.
19. Stern JM, Yiee J, Park S. Safety and efficacy of ureteral access sheaths. J Endourol. 2007; 21(2):119–23.
20. Auge BK, Pietrow PK, Lallas CD, et al. Ureteral access sheath provides protection against elevated renal pressures during routine flexible ureteroscopic stone manipulation. J Endourol. 2004;18(1):33–6.
21. Lallas CD, Auge BK, Raj GV, et al. Laser Doppler flowmetric determination of ureteral blood flow; after ureteral access sheath placement. J Endourol. 2002;16(8):583–90.
22. Monga M, Gawlik A, Durfee W. Systematic evaluation of ureteral access sheaths. Urology. 2004;63(5):834–6.
23. Monga M, Best S, Venkatesh R, et al. Prospective randomized comparison of 2 ureteral access sheaths during flexible retrograde ureteroscopy. J Urol. 2004;172(2):572–3.

24. Hendlin K, Weiland D, Monga M. Impact of irrigation systems on stone migration. J Endourol. 2008;22(3):453–8.
25. Elashry OM, Tawfik AM. Preventing stone retropulsion during intracorporeal lithotripsy. Nat Rev Urol. 2012;9(12):691–8.
26. Ahmed M, Pedro RN, Kieley S, et al. Systematic evaluation of ureteral occlusion devices: insertion, deployment, stone migration, and extraction. Urology. 2009;73(5):976–80.
27. Knudsen B. Flexible ureteroscopy: holmium: YAG laser and optical fibers. In: Monga M, editor. Ureteroscopy: indications, instrumentation, and technique. New York: Springer Science+Business Media; 2013. p. 161–8.
28. Bagley DH, Kuo RL, Zeltser IS. An update on ureteroscopic instrumentation for the treatment of urolithiasis. Curr Opin Urol. 2004;14(2):99–106.
29. Leveillee RJ, Lobik L. Intracorporeal lithotripsy: which modality is best? Curr Opin Urol. 2003;13(3):249–53.
30. Miller J, Stoller M. Intracorporeal lithotripsy: electrohydraulic, pneumatic, and ultrasonic. In: Monga M, editor. Ureteroscopy: indications, instrumentation, and technique. New York: Springer Science+Business Media; 2013. p. 149–60.

Chapter 12
Tips and Tricks in the Treatment of Ureteral Stones

David Leavitt, Sammy Elsamra, David Hoenig, and Zeph Okeke

Introduction

As with any surgical treatment, the successful management of patients with ureteral stones relies on both proper patient selection and sound surgical principles. The purpose of this chapter is to highlight many of the most useful tips and tricks of SWL and URS when used to treat ureteral stones. Ureteral stones can be managed in a variety of ways. Medical expulsive therapy (MET), shockwave lithotripsy (SWL), ureteroscopy (URS), percutaneous renal access with antegrade ureteroscopy, laparoscopic or robotic ureterolithotomy and open ureterolithotomy are all various techniques that have been used to treat ureteral stones. In the early 1980s SWL was introduced and drastically reduced the need for open ureterolithotomy. Over the ensuing decades semirigid and then flexible ureteroscopy became more widely utilized with the miniaturization of the ureteroscopes and working instruments, and with the increasing dissemination of surgical technique necessary for safe ureteroscopy. Indeed, in areas where SWL and URS equipment is readily available, open ureteral stone surgery is only rarely undertaken.

Shockwave Lithotripsy

The use of shockwave energy to fracture kidney and ureteral stones was initially performed in humans in the early 1980s in Germany. The Dornier HM3 lithotripter was first produced and distributed in 1983 and the United States Food and Drug Administration approved its use for urinary stones in 1984. Shockwave lithotripsy

D. Leavitt • S. Elsamra • D. Hoenig • Z. Okeke (✉)
The Smith Institute for Urology, Hofstra North Shore Long Island Jewish School of Medicine, 450 Lakeville Road, New Hyde Park, NY 11042, USA
e-mail: dleavitt@nshs.edu; selsamra@nshs.edu; dhoenig@nshs.edu; zokeke@nshs.edu

S.R. Patel, S.Y. Nakada (eds.), *Ureteral Stone Management: A Practical Approach*, DOI 10.1007/978-3-319-08792-4_12

revolutionized urinary stone management because of its noninvasive nature, relatively high effectiveness and ease of treatment. Over the last 40 years, considerable experience has been gained regarding the nuances of SWL and this information can be used to improve patient selection for shockwave lithotripsy and to improve the outcomes for a given patient who is undergoing SWL.

There are a number of factors that should be considered when deciding if SWL is the preferred treatment modality for a patient, and these include patient features, stone characteristics and technical factors. Though many of the stone characteristics cannot be changed, many of the technical and some of the patient-specific factors can be modified to improve success rates and reduce morbidity associated with SWL. This section highlights the tips and tricks to treating ureteral stones with SWL.

Technical Factors

One of the easiest, and most important, aspects of SWL treatment that can be modified is the rate at which shockwaves are generated, or the shockwave firing rate. Good level I evidence exists showing that a slower firing rate, rather than a faster one, provides better stone clearance [1, 2]. In fact, a rate between 60 and 90 shocks per minute appears to be best and has been recommended as the preferred rate by the AUA/EAU guidelines. A slower firing rate may also cause less renal tissue damage as fewer overall shocks are necessary for stone fragmentation, but is frequently associated with a slightly longer operative time [3].

Animal studies have shown SWL induces renal tissue and vascular damage which appears to be dose-dependent, and may be reduced by altering the amplitude of energy delivered during SWL and the rate at which the energy is increased over the course of a treatment session. Voltage escalation, or voltage stepping as it is also known, involves a stepwise increase in energy settings as the shockwave treatment session progresses. Some data suggest a slow or delayed voltage escalation may be associated with less renal damage compared to an immediate ramping up of the energy, so long as the time difference between lower amplitude and higher amplitude shockwaves is approximately 3–4 min [4]. It is controversial whether or not voltage escalation improves stone free rates (SFR), as some studies report it does while others report no effect.

Shockwaves are reflected by air or air-bubbles within the coupling medium. In fact, a 20–40 % decrease in stone breakage has been seen when as little as 2 % of the coupling interface is covered with air pockets [5, 6]. Thus, another simple strategy to improve SWL success is by optimizing the coupling between the patient and lithotripter. Choosing a coupling medium such as oil or gel is favored. The coupling medium should be applied generously and directly to the patient's skin or shockwave head as a large dollop and allowed to disperse via contact between the skin and treatment head. If instead, the coupling medium is rubbed onto the skin or shockwave treatment head, additional air pockets are introduced along the coupling surface resulting in less effective shockwave transmission.

Another important factor affecting SWL success is ensuring the F2 focal point remains over the stone as much as possible during lithotripsy. The kidneys and to a lesser extent the proximal ureter are subject to spatial variation with respiratory excursions. Some data suggest up to 40 % of shocks during a given treatment session may actually miss the stone because of stone movement with respirations [7, 8]. One way to minimize this is with general anesthesia, thereby allowing for the use of a lower tidal volume and less respiratory-induced stone movement. Furthermore, general anesthesia reduces overall patient movement. This is advantageous as increased patient movement interferes with optimal coupling by introducing air pockets between the patient and lithotripter treatment head.

As a general rule, ureteral stenting is not advised prior to SWL of ureteral stones in the absence of another indication for placing a ureteral stent. Similarly, stone manipulation or pushback into the renal pelvis does not improve SFR and should be discouraged [9]. In the past, the placement of ureteral stents or relocating a ureteral stone into the renal pelvis was thought to improve stone fragmentation by increasing the aqueous micro-environment around the stone allowing for better shockwave transmittance. In addition, ureteral stenting was thought to improve stone passage rates and minimize post-SWL complications such as steinstrasse.

However, mounting prospective randomized evidence suggests stents are associated with increased suprapubic pain, dysuria, hematuria and lower urinary tract symptoms, yet have no appreciable influence on SFR and may actually worsen it [10]. As such the AUA/EAU guidelines now recommend against ureteral stent placement during SWL [1]. One caveat, of course, is that ureteral stents should be used in patients with solitary kidneys.

Fluoroscopy and ultrasound are the two modalities presently used to visualize stones during SWL. Unfortunately, ultrasound is rarely helpful in localizing ureteral stones. Fluoroscopy can be problematic if stones are radiolucent (i.e. predominately uric acid stones), the patient is morbidly obese, or if the stone is projected over a bony prominence such as the pelvic bones or vertebral transverse processes. In these cases where stones are poorly visualized for whatever reason, an intravenous pyelogram (IVP) or retrograde pyelogram (RGP) can be used to better target the stone.

Similar to air, skeletal bones impede shockwave transmission. This becomes particularly important for mid and distal ureteral stones as the bony pelvis can attenuate shockwave delivery in these locations. Analogously, the transverse processes may interfere with shockwave delivery to proximal ureteral stones. Repositioning patients in the prone position can improve SWL effectiveness for mid and distal ureteral stones. Another option is to modestly angle (20–30°) patients into a rotated-supine (for proximal ureteral stones) or rotated-prone (for mid and distal ureteral stones) position which may further minimize shock-wave attenuation from surrounding bony structures [11].

A number of studies have demonstrated the beneficial effects of alpha-blockers given to patients immediately following ureteral stone treatment with SWL. Alpha-blockers can increase SFRs, accelerate stone passage after SWL fragmentation, and reduce postoperative analgesic requirements [1, 12, 13]. Most alpha-blockers have a good safety profile and should be used unless contraindicated.

The value of an experienced shockwave lithotripsy technologist should not be underestimated, as many mobile shockwave units are now utilized. A good technologist can assist with proper patient positioning on a given machine, can facilitate stone localization at the F2 focal zone, can help reduce radiation exposure, and can simplify device troubleshooting when problems arise.

Stone Characteristics

Stone Composition

Not all stones are equally susceptible to fragmentation by SWL and the expected size of the fragments generated also differs depending on stone composition. In general, cystine, calcium hydrogen phosphate and calcium oxalate monohydrate stones are more resistant to adequate fragmentation with SWL than other stone types [14]. Interestingly, calcium oxalate monohydrate and cystine stones frequently produce larger fragments that are less likely to spontaneously pass and may increase the risk for subsequent obstruction and steinstrasse. Stone attenuation as measured by Hounsfield units (HU) also impacts on SWL success. Higher HU are associated with worse fragmentation and more SWL treatment failures, and HU >900–1,000 appear to be a common cutoff between good and poor fragmentation in many studies [15]. Taken together, SWL should be approached with caution in patients with a history of cystine, calcium hydrogen phosphate and calcium oxalate monohydrate stones, and in stones with HU >900–1,000.

Stone Location

The location of a stone also has a role in the treatment efficacy of SWL. Proximal ureteral stones tend to be easier to target than mid and distal ureteral stones, and for this reason SWL is often preferentially employed for proximal ureteral stones and provides good SFRs of approximately 80 %. Stones in the mid ureter are more challenging to visualize given the sacrum which can confound fluoroscopic or ultrasonic targeting, while distal ureteral stones can be difficult to localize when pelvic phleboliths are in close proximity. The pelvic bones can also impede shockwave transmission. Placing patients prone, or into a rotated-prone position reduces bony pelvis interference with shockwave delivery. This can be combined with an IVP or RPG if necessary to enhance stone targeting. With these strategies, SFRs of approximately 75 % have been reported for mid ureteral stones, and SFRs as high as 90 % have been reported for distal ureteral stones treated with SWL [16, 17].

Stone Size

Stone fragmentation and SWL success decrease as stone size increases. At any given ureteral location, SFRs are higher for stones <1 cm compared to stones >1 cm [1]. Moreover, many reports suggest stones greater than 10 mm are associated with significantly lower SFRs and require more treatment sessions than ureteroscopy, and this is true for both distal and proximal ureteral stones [1]. As such SWL appears best suited to tackle ureteral stone burdens less than approximately 1 cm.

Patient Features

Skin to stone distance has been shown to impact SWL success with decreasing SFR achieved as skin-to-stone distance increases. This may be the result of a combination of factors including shockwave attenuation as it passes through more tissue to reach the stone and poorer imaging quality and stone targeting as Xrays are similarly degraded as they pass through the additional tissue. Many studies have found stark reductions in stone clearance when skin-to-stone distance was great than 9–10 cm [15].

When employing SWL in morbidly obese individuals, various strategies can improve SFRs including use of abdominal compression or utilizing an extended shockwave blast pathway [18]. Abdominal compression mechanically reduces the skin-to-stone distance. An extended shockwave blast pathway creates high shock wave pressures at a focus past F2, delivering more energy to stones outside of the F2 zone. When employing these techniques, realize higher total energy delivery is often necessary and SWL machines that generate the largest peak pressures with the longest focal length work best.

Successful SWL also depends on proper patient positioning. This can be a challenge in patients with skeletal deformities, significant contractures and certain malrotated and ectopic kidneys. Careful review of preoperative cross-sectional imaging is very helpful in these situations and can help determine if a reasonable shockwave blast path exists from skin to stone without intervening air or bone.

Ureteroscopy

Ureteroscopy has undergone significant advances over the past several years. Rigid ureteroscopes are rarely used and have been replaced with semirigid and flexible ureteroscopes. Ureteroscopes have evolved to include smaller overall calibers, larger working channels, active and dual deflection in flexible ureteroscopes, and improved optics. Along with similar improvements in ancillary equipment for ureteroscopy (wires, laser fibers, baskets, etc.), the role for ureteroscopy in the treatment of ureteral and renal pathology has expanded and despite considerably increased utilization, complication rates during ureteroscopy have sharply decreased. The purpose of this section is to highlight some of the tips and tricks associated with ureteroscopy for the treatment of ureteral stones.

General Recommendations

Ureteral Access

Safely and properly accessing the ureter for ureteroscopy is critical to optimizing ureteroscopy outcomes and reducing attendant risks. With the miniaturization of flexible and semirigid ureteroscopes, often with tip diameters as small as 6–8Fr, many ureters and ureteral stones can be adequately accessed and treated without dilation of the ureteral orifice or ureter. Nonetheless, in certain cases there is still a role for actively dilating the ureteral orifice or a ureteral stricture, if encountered.

A distinction should be made between a ureteral stricture and a ureteral spasm or physiologically narrow ureter. A ureteral stricture is often associated with proximal hydroureteronephrosis and urothelium around the strictured site will appear white and more pale than surrounding healthy urothelium. In contrast, a physiologically narrow ureter or ureteral spams, should not have proximal hydroureteronephrosis and there should be no apparent changes in the involved urothelium.

As stones can often migrate between the time of presentation and the time of surgery, it is prudent to assess for stone migration prior to ureteral dilation. Performing a gentle retrograde pyelogram accomplishes this goal and provides additional useful anatomic information. Another option is to perform semirigid ureteroscopy prior to ureteral dilation and prior to placement of a ureteral access sheath. This should help avoid inappropriate ureteral dilation at the site of the stone which can cause injury to the ureteral wall or stone perforation through the ureteral wall.

Ureteral dilation should be done over a guidewire. Numerous dilators exist, with the goal of each to dilater the ureter as minimally and with the least amount of applied force as possible to accomplish the task. Balloon dilators come in a variety of sizes with 15–18Fr diameter appropriate for most ureters. Ensure the balloon is filled with radiopaque fluid during inflation so it may be visualized fluoroscopically during inflation (Fig. 12.1). If dilation of more than just the ureteral orifice is considered, dilating in a proximal-to-distal direction is safest. Dilating pressures up to 12–14 atmospheres are generally safe, and higher pressures should be done with care. Proximal ureteral balloon dilation should be done cautiously as the proximal ureter is most susceptible to perforation and avulsion injury.

Dilation may also be carried out with small caliber (10–14Fr) ureteral dilators, with a 10Fr dual lumen catheter (which are often 6Fr at the tip), with 8/10Fr coaxial dilators and with the 10Fr tip of the Amplatz Renal fasical dilator set. The internal obturator of a ureteral access sheath can also serve as a ureteral dilator if initial attempts at placement of the combined ureteral access sheath-internal dilator meet resistance. Ureteral dilation is often best accomplished over a stiffer wire (i.e. Amplatz Superstiff wire) as it helps prevent buckling of the access sheath. Copious lubrication should be used with any dilator to facilitate ureteral passage, and caution must be used upon passage of any ureteral dilator as aggressive advancement may result in ureteral injury.

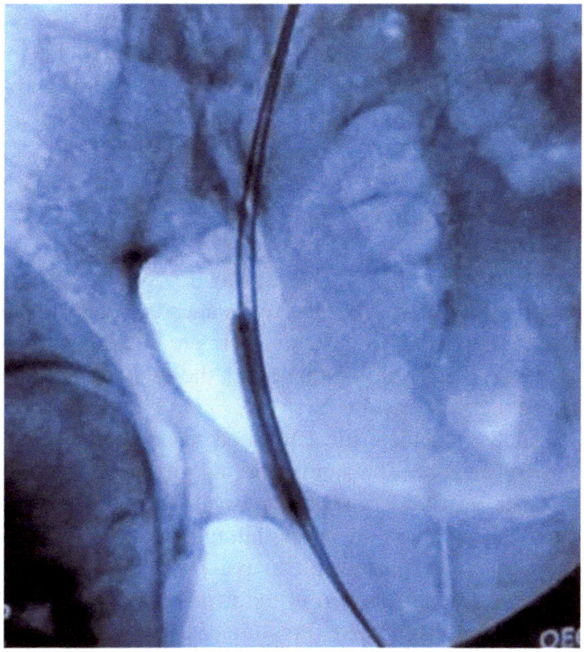

Fig. 12.1 Fluoroscopic image of balloon dilation of distal right ureter

In addition, performing semirigid ureteroscopy prior to any planned flexible ureteroscopy can also serve to dilate the ureter and ease passage of subsequent instruments. Despite these tactics, if the ureter remains too narrow or does not easily accommodate the ureteroscope or ureteral access sheath, then placement of an indwelling ureteral stent for at least 1 week can allow for passive ureteral dilation. Thereafter, subsequent attempts to access the ureter are frequently successful.

Furthermore, not all ureteroscopes are the same. Size of the flexible ureteroscope is an important parameter with regard to access. While digital flexible ureteroscopes have recently seen increased utilization due to clear improvements in visualization, they are often greater in diameter than analog ones. Despite a difference of less than 2Fr in diameter, this difference was found to be enough to require a significantly greater proportion of ureteral access sheath utilization [19].

In cases of tortuous ureters, the combination of an angled wire and angled ureteral catheter can negotiate almost any series of ureteral twists and turns. The use of different caliber wires (0.038″, 0.025″, and 0.018″) can be helpful as well. In addition, if initial attempts to advance a non-hydrophylic wire (Bentson wire) are met with resistance, then changing to a hydrophilic wire (i.e., Glidewire or Sensor wire) can ease wire placement. Once the wire has been successfully placed into the renal pelvis, exchanging it for a stiffer wire (i.e. Amplatz Superstiff) through a ureteral catheter will better straighten out the ureter and simplify subsequent ureteroscopy attempts.

Ectopic ureteral orifice location, such as with cross-trigonal ureteral reimplants and renal transplant ureters, can pose a distinct challenge to adequately access for successful ureteroscopy. Gentle balloon dilation with subsequent placement of a stiff guidewire can be helpful and has been reported with success [20].

Poor Visualization

Several parameters may be adjusted to optimize visualization during ureteroscopy. The first of which is proper focus ahead of placement of the ureteroscope into the ureter. In non-digital systems, there are two items to focus; the scope itself and the camera, whereas in digital scopes the digital chip is located within the scope and hence focus is singular.

Another factor critical to good visualization during ureteroscopy is adequate flow of irrigant. The small working channels of most ureteroscopes and the long distance over which irrigation travels from source to ureteroscope creates significant resistance to flow necessitating some form or pressurized irrigation. A variety of instruments are available to assist with this task.

Pressure bags applied to the irrigation source are one option and are reusable, and hence cost-effective. Pressure can be modified by opening or closing the inflow valve near the ureteroscope. Hand pumps controlled either by the surgeon or by an assistant (i.e., Single-Action-Pump or Pathfinder) are alternatives. These systems are single-use and pressurize only a small volume of irrigant but do so at surgeon desired intervals and allow for temporary generation of higher pressures than those created with pressure bags. Foot-pedal activated pumps can also be utilized, but can be cumbersome if also using a lithotripter foot pedal. With any of these systems, care must be taken to avoid retropulsion of the stone.

Ensure there is no kinking along the irrigation tubing and eliminate air bubble introduction within the line to avoid air locks. If visualization is poor with an instrument through the working channel, consider using a smaller diameter instrument. In most instances in which a laser fiber is indicated a smaller size fiber between 200 and 365 μm will be sufficient. Similarly, many of the new stone baskets are of smaller caliber (1.5–1.9Fr) and provide adequate basket size, grasping strength and durability.

Sometimes during ureteroscopy a significant degree of light glare and artifact is present and can obscure the view. This can be noticed in particular with some of the contemporary digital and high definition optical systems. Decreasing the light source intensity or brightness helps minimize glare by decreasing the light reflectivity from the urothelium.

Patient Positioning

The ureter does not follow a straight course from kidney to bladder, and a couple of positioning strategies can facilitate ureteroscopy. The lithotomy position is preferred for routine ureteroscopy as the surgeon has ease access to the urethra and can ergonomically pass instruments along the same axis as the general course of the ureter. Reducing the degree of hip flexion and slightly abducting the hip ipsilateral to the side of the ureteral stone can straighten the course of the ureter as it travels across the psoas muscle and ease ureteroscope passage in this area [21].

Always be cognizant of frozen lower extremity joints, as it may not be possible to safely position the patient in such a way as to easily accommodate rigid or semi-rigid instruments. In these cases, flexible cystoscopes and ureteroscopes are necessary. In addition, flexible instruments may be necessary in patients with considerable pelvic scar tissue, such as those with a history of prior pelvic surgery, pelvic radiation, and pelvic malignancies.

Stone Basketing

One of the most common causes for iatrogenic ureteral injury during stone surgery occurs at the time of stone basketing, and usually results when attempting to extract a stone or fragment that is too large. Myriad baskets exist for stone retrieval, and as a general rule tipless baskets should be used, rather than baskets with tips, as they are less likely to directly perforate the ureter. When extracting a stone or fragment it is important to keep the basketed stone close to the tip of the ureteroscope and in direct vision throughout. If too large a gap exists between the basketed stone and ureteroscope tip, the ureteral wall can catch in this space and become injured or intussuscepted during stone removal.

Minimal resistance should be encountered during stone basket extraction, and the basket should never be forced or yanked. When an area of resistance is encountered, adjusting the stone's orientation within the ureter or basket should be attempted. This is accomplished by opening the basket approximately half way and gently manipulating the basket proximally and distally, side-to-side, or rotationally. This allows the long axis of the stone to naturally realign with the long axis of the ureter. Thereafter, the basket can again be fully closed to secured the stone in the most favorable orientation and reattempt basket extraction.

Occasionally it becomes difficult or impossible to disengage a basket from a large stone fragment or fragments. In these instances, a few tactics can be tried. If there is room to pass a small laser fiber (i.e. 200 μm) alongside the basket, a small amount of energy applied directly to the stone is often sufficient to fragment the stone further and allow for basket disengagement. Alternatively, the laser can be used to cut one of the prongs of the basket, but one must ensure no basket pieces are left behind as these can serve as a nidus for further stone nucleation and growth.

Another option is to disassemble the basket at its handle, as some baskets have a screw mechanism that will free the handle from the rest of the basket. As a next step, withdraw the ureteroscope leaving the stone and basket in place within the ureter. Then reintroduce the ureteroscope alongside the basket and fragment the stone with laser. The basket can then be removed and a new one reinserted through the working channel of the ureteroscope.

Impacted Ureteral Stones

Impacted ureteral stone often present a challenge. They can be associated with an intense inflammatory reaction and ureteral edema around the impaction site which can obscure vision and interfere with safely positioning the laser or other lithotripsy fiber onto the stone. Once a guidewire has been safely advanced past the stone to the pelvicalyceal system, gentle attempts to maneuver the stone proximally into the often more dilated and non-inflammed ureter can be attempted. This provides additional space for irrigation and safe stone lithotripsy. Again, this should be done carefully and with only minimal force.

If you cannot pass the stone with a wire, options must be carefully assessed. In experience hands, an attempt to perform ureteroscopy to the stone and laser it without a safety wire in placed can be considered. With this approach, judicious laser use is recommended until the stone disimpacts, after which reattempts at wire placement should ensue. However, ureteroscopy and laser lithotripsy in the absence of a safety wire can be associated with significant complications, and have a nephrostomy tube or antegrade ureteral stent placed are reasonable alternatives.

If this stone does not easily move proximally, then judicious lithotripsy of the distal most aspect of the impacted stone is recommended. Dusting the distal edge of impacted ureteral calculi should minimizing the creation of large fragments and can be accomplished by using high frequency and low energy settings of the laser generator. Sometimes rotating the ureteroscope clockwise or counterclockwise along its long axis will change the position at which the lithotripter fiber contacts the stone and can be particularly helpful if a portion of the stone is covered by edematous urothelium. Then once the stone becomes disimpacted, it can be manipulated proximally to the more open and dilated ureter.

Preventing Proximal Stone Migration

The use of anti-retropulsion devices within the ureter can help reduce the proximal migration of stones and improve stone free rates. The Stone Cone (Boston Scientific, Natick, MA) and the NTrap (Cook Medical, Bloomington, IN) are two such devices, however each is attached to its own additional guidewire, which narrows the working space within the ureter, and comes with an additional disposable instrument cost.

To avoid the need for an additional wire, thermoactive liquid gels have been utilized and are deposited just proximal to the ureteral stone thereby creating a temporary barrier to proximal stone migration (BackStop liquid gel, Boston Scientific, Natick, MA). Surgical lubrication has also been described as a suitable and cheap agent for preventing proximal migration of fragments [22].

When the Laser Fails

It is reasonable to have a backup plan should the laser fail. If no substitute laser is available, consider pneumatic lithotripsy as an alternative (i.e. EMS Swiss Lithoclast or Olympus LUS 2). Though laser has a better safety profile, intraureteral pneumatic lithotripsy has been well documented as a viable technique with acceptably low complication rates [23]. Given the rigidity of the pneumatic probes, this is only feasible with a semirigid ureteroscope with a straight-entry working channel and offset lens. Keep in mind, ureteral stent insertion and returning for completion ureteroscopy at a later date is sometimes the most prudent option.

Medical Expulsive Therapy

Alpha blockers have been shown to increase SFR after ureteroscopy for ureteral stones [24]. In addition, alpha blockers help alleviate ureteral stent symptoms, pain, sexual life symptoms and overall quality of life following ureteroscopy [25]. As such if there are no contraindications, alpha blockers are reasonable to prescribe following ureteroscopy.

Semirigid Ureteroscopy

Semirigid ureteroscopy is the preferred treatment modality for most distal ureteral stones. In some patients, semirigid ureteroscopes can be safely advanced into the proximal ureter and renal pelvis. Compared to flexible ureteroscopes, semirigid ureteroscopes are more steady and maneuverable within the distal ureter and generally offers better optical quality than most flexible ureteroscopes. Furthermore, semirigid ureteroscopes usually have larger working channels allowing for improved irrigation even when using larger instruments and multiple instruments.

When performing semirigid ureteroscopy, the intial step is to place a safety wire. The safety wire allows for ureteral stenting should any difficulty arise during ureteroscopy. The safety wire also assists with ureteral access. Floppy tip, hydrophilic wires are recommended as the initial wire most likely to advance easily and least likely to perforate the ureter when navigating around a ureteral stone. Once positioned in the renal pelvis, these wires can be exchanged to a stiffer wire (i.e. Amplatz SuperStiff) through a small ureteral catheter (as previously discussed, a stiffer wire can better straighten the ureter).

Once the safety wire is placed, access into the ureter can be achieved through a number of different techniques. Passing the ureteroscope directly under the wire toward the ureteral orifice helps further tent the orifice open allowing the scope to pass under the wire and into the ureter (Fig. 12.2). Very small controlled movements should be used with the ureteroscope as readjusting even a few millimeters can be the difference between entering and missing the ureter.

If the ureteral orifice cannot be entered by passing the ureteroscope underneath the wire, try riding on top of the wire and using the scope to push down on the wire just as it enters the ureter. This can allow entry into the ureter when advancing below the wire fails.

If these techniques are unsuccessful, using a two-wire, or "railroad," technique should be tried next (Fig. 12.3). Once the safety wire is in place, pass a separate wire through the working channel of the ureteroscope and intubate the ureteral orifice

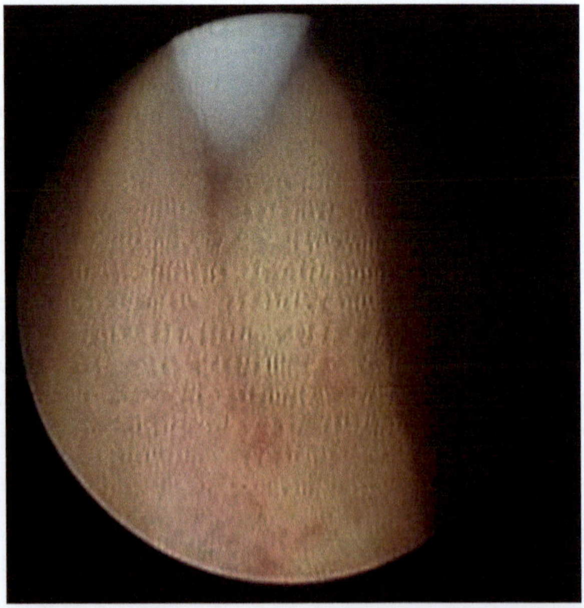

Fig. 12.2 Passing semirigid ureteroscope directly underneath guidewire that is tenting open ureter

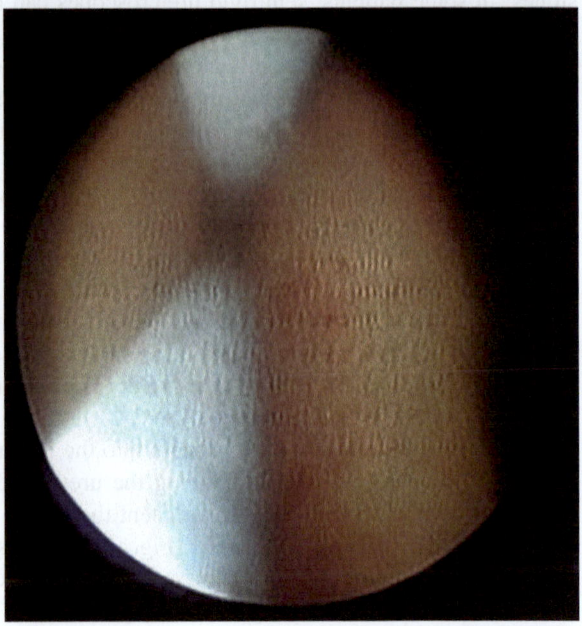

Fig. 12.3 "Railroad" technique for accessing the ureter, using one guide wire to tent open the ureter and a second guide wire passed through the working channel of the ureteroscope

with the new wire. Next rotate the semirigid ureteroscope such that the beak of the scope is aligned between the two wires and advance the scope through the ureteral orifice in this manner. A stone basket, rather than a second guidewire, may be used to perform the railroad technique, but care should be taken as the stone baskets are more likely to kink and have a greater tendency to perforate the urothelium.

Once in the ureter, the wire through the working channel of the ureteroscope can be used in a similar fashion to negotiate past any additional narrow areas. Alternatively, partially opening a stone basket just in front of the tip of the ureteroscope often straightens this segment of ureter and allows for segmental advancement of ureteroscope. Another option is to softly manipulate the safety wire in or out by approximately 1 cm. This can further straighten out areas of ureteral kinking and reduce areas of ureteral redundancy. Contemporary semirigid ureteroscopes have a beveled beak and this feature can be exploited by rotating the handle of the ureteroscope clockwise or counterclockwise. In this manner, the beak of the ureteroscope can be aligned better to the contour of the ureter improving the ability to safely navigate some of the narrower portions of the ureter such as the pelvic brim.

Ensuring the bladder is mostly empty simplifies distal ureteroscopy by eliminating the posterolateral angulation of the ureter that occurs with a distended bladder. Some advocate for placing a small 10–14Fr urethral catheter alongside the semirigid ureteroscope when performing ureteroscopy to ensure continuous bladder emptying.

Semirigid ureteroscopy can be difficult in men with large prostates and associated J-hooking of the distal ureter. Balloon dilation of the distal ureter and placement of a stiff safety wire can help straighten the ureter. In some instances using a peel-away ureteral access sheath can facilitate re-entry into the distal ureter if multiple passes are anticipated. Note that most fixed-length ureteral access sheaths are too long to use for this technique. Also, after ureteral stone lithotripsy, good inspection of the distal most aspect of the ureter just before the intramural ureter is important as stone fragments will often collect here and have a difficult time passing spontaneously given the J-hooking of the ureter.

Flexible Ureteroscopy

Considerable technological advances in flexible ureteroscopy, and increased exposure to cases during urological residency, have contributed to its increasing utilization. Flexible ureteroscopy has utility in the surveillance and treatment of ureteral stricture disease, upper tract urothelial tumors, and urolithiasis. Indeed, even staghorn calculi can be treated with flexible ureteroscopy and laser lithotripsy. While such indications are beyond the scope of this chapter, they highlight the expanding role of ureteroscopy within the field of urology. The use of flexible ureteroscopy for the treatment of ureteral stones has been previously described in this text and as such some advice may be mentioned in both chapters.

Indication

Flexible ureteroscopy for ureteral stones is typically limited to cases not amenable to safe approach with the semi-rigid URS. One indication for flexible ureteroscopy is the proximal ureter (identified as the region of the ureter above the iliac vessels). The utilization of a flexible ureteroscope for such stones is often required for safe access. Ureteral angulation above the vessels may preclude the safe usage of a semi-rigid ureteroscope. Further, flexible ureteroscopy may be beneficial in cases of distal ureteral stone in patients with large prostates which might limit the use of a semi-rigid ureterosocpe. Similarly in patients with a history of cross-trigonal ureteral ureteroneocystostomy, flexible ureteroscopy may overcome angulation associated with such distal ureters via an orthotopic or percutaneous transvesical approach [20].

Access

The use of the flexible ureteroscope within the ureter is dependent upon appropriate and safe insertion. We favor clearance of the distal ureter, either radiographically or visually with antecedent passage of a semi-rigid ureteroscope prior to advancement of a flexible ureteroscope up the ureter. This will allow the surgeon to assess not only the caliber of the ureter, hence permitting a judgement as to whether or not it will accommodate the flexible ureteroscope, but also ensure a clear distal ureter free of stone fragments or ureteral strictures which may complicate flexible ureteroscopy. This is particularly important as visualization of the ureterovseical junction (UVJ) with the flexible ureteroscope may be limited in light of the two methods for its introduction into the ureter.

The scope is advanced in one of two ways up the ureter. The first is the two wire technique, whereby both a safety and working wire are advanced up the ureter under fluoroscopic guidance. With the safety wire secured to the drapes, the flexible ureteroscope is advanced over the working wire to the point of the ureteral stone. Note the working wire in these cases must have a floppy or soft distal tip to avoid scope damage when advancing over the wire. Care must be taken to keep back tension on the wire and to advance the scope under fluoroscopic guidance as buckling of the scope may occur and excess scope and wire may be advanced into a loop within the bladder.

By virtue of the fact that the working channel is on the posterior aspect of the scope (eccentric-parallel axis) and the wire may be tented up on the anterior aspect of the UVJ, the flexible ureteroscope may buckle at this interface. An easy way to correct for this is to rotate the flexible ureteroscope 180° such that the lower profile portion of the scope is anterior (where the wire is tented up); this allows for the tented ureteral orifice to accommodate the major axis of the scope, posteriorly.

The other method for access into the ureter with the flexible ureteroscope is to utilize a ureteral access sheath. While there are many different types of ureteral access sheaths (coaxial obturator and sheath vs balloon dilated sheath) and variation in diameter and length, once placed they allow for facile passage of the flexible ureteroscope through its lumen into the ureter, bypassing the urethra, intravesical portion, UVJ, and the distal ureter. Ureteral access sheath use has been associated with shorter operative times, less ureteroscope damage, less intrarenal pressure and improved visualization. Despite some concern initially with ureteral access sheaths potentially predisposing to ureteral strictures, the available evidence refutes this concern. Details regarding coaxial and balloon dilating ureteral access sheaths are outlined in other sections of this text.

In the setting of a ureteral stricture (proximal to the UVJ), advancement of a flexible ureteroscope may be difficult due to lack of rigidity and control at the tip of the scope. The utilization of a working wire passed through the scope and advanced beyond the stricture, may allow for tenting of the stricture and provide rigidity at the tip of the flexible scope to prevent buckling and allow for passage. Further, a stiffer wire may provide increased tensile force to resist such buckling. In general, keeping the extracorporeal portion of the ureteroscope as straight as possible facilitates intracorporeal ureteroscope advancement and deflection capabilities, and should be kept in mind when having trouble advancing the ureteroscope.

Laser, Basket, or Both?

Once a stone is visualized decision must be made for either basket-extraction or fragmentation. We favor basket extraction for stones whenever possible, as it will decrease the stone burden and provide a specimen for biochemical analysis. The critical question, however, is to what size stones can be safely extracted. Surgeon judgment is important, but may be unreliable. Bin et al. demonstrated that along with stone size, a previously stented ureteral system were the only significant factors predictive of mitigating the need for ureteral dilation ahead of stone basket extraction [26]. Further, in a review of nearly 850 patients, stone diameter of 8 mm or greater was associated with unfavorable outcomes [27]. Hence, we consider basket extraction only up to this size and in the presence of useful dilation. Otherwise, we attempt fragmentation of larger stones into a few stones, each smaller than 8 mm to facilitate extraction. However, surgeon estimation of stone size utilizing endoscopic visualization may be limited [28].

Laser fragmentation is a mainstay for the treatment of ureteral and renal stones utilizing the flexible ureteroscope. We favor the utilization of a 200 μm diameter laser fiber through the flexible ureteroscope it will impede flow less than a 365 μm fiber (flow is proportional to diameter to the fourth power per Poiseuille's Law). While not pertinent to the treatment of a ureteral stone, the 200 μm fiber will also hinder flexion within the scope the least, allowing for usage of the same fiber for a renal stone or in case of retropulsion.

Laser fibers may be utilized to fragment or to "dust" the stone. Fragmentation is typically performed with high energy and low frequency whereas dusting is utilizing low energy and high frequency. The main determinant, in our estimate, for which setting ought to be utilized is the density of the stone. We favor dusting softer stones and fragmenting (with subsequent basket extraction) of harder stones [29].

With repeated stone basket extraction, it cannot be stressed enough that the risk of ureteral injury and its sequelae (stricture, need for additional surgical procedures, renal loss) are serious, albeit rare, complications. In any cases where a question exists, fragmentation rather than intact stone extraction is safer.

Stone baskets come in various types and sizes. Whereas some larger helical baskets may be utilized with a semirigid ureteroscope, their large lumens and stiff core prevent reasonable use within flexible ureteroscopes. We favor the use of a tipless nitinol basket or grasper. Commonly, a 3-Fr basket is available and is often utilized but may impede flow, particularly if the flexible ureteroscope is deflected. Even with the use of a 1.9Fr basket, flow within most flexible ureteroscopes decreases significantly. Utilization of a ureteral access sheath is preferred when basket extraction is intended as it allows facile access to the proximal ureter without the need for wire replacement and guidance for scope reinsertion. Should a stone be too large for the sheath, but not too large for the ureter, both stone and sheath may be extracted in unison; with subsequent replacement of the ureteral access sheath if needed.

Percutaneous Antegrade Nephrolithotomy and Ureteroscopy

Antegrade flexible ureteroscopy may be performed during a percutaneous nephrolithotomy (PCNL) when the patient has ureteral stones, either present on pre-op imaging or if there is concern for stone migration down the ureter during the PCNL. It may also be performed in such cases when retrograde ureteroscopy is not facile or feasible; such as in a patient with a urinary diversion or complex distal ureteral anatomy. It may be beneficial to consider antgrade antegrade flexible ureteroscopy for cases of large impacted stone in the distal ureter. To this end, we recommend access via a posterior calyx that allows for the minimal flexion at the UPJ. When anticipating multiple passes into the ureter, then consider placing a ureteral access in an antegrade fashion to facilitate ureteroscope re-entry into the ureter and to help protect the UPJ. Also, if limited work is anticipated within the kidney, then tract dilation may be to a lesser extent than with PCNL and allows for smaller access sheath use.

We find that the surgeon may retain significant control of the flexible scope if there is no additional deflection located high in the scope; let alone with two possible deflections and instruments placed within the working channel. Further, flexible ureteroscopey may be performed with a flexible cystoscope as often the obstructed ureter is dilated and can accommodate a 16Fr scope; this allows for greater visualization and workability with often difficult stones. Additionally, when fragmented, such impacted distal stones may not require retrieval but rather may be pushed beyond the ureteral orfice for clearance. Ultimately, an antegrade pyeoloureterogram, in addition to direct visualization, is recommended to ensure there is no evidence of obstruction or extravasation at the end of every antegrade flexible ureteroscopy.

Conclusion

A variety of treatment options exist for ureteral stones, with ureteroscopy and shockwave lithotripsy utilized most frequently when this technology is available. Percutaneous nephrolithotomy and antegrade ureteroscopy are reserved for cases when SWL or ureteroscopy have failed or when dictated by anatomic considerations.

Just as no ureteral stone patient is exactly the same, no treatment session, no matter the modality, follows the exact same sequence of events from patient to patient. New and different challenges are encountered with each case necessitating on-the-job troubleshooting. The tips and tricks detailed in this chapter represent the collective experience gained over many years from a myriad of urologists. The hope is that these tips and tricks will be incorporated to improve the safety, outcomes and value of treatment delivered to patients with ureteral stones.

Ureteral Stone Treatment Tips and Tricks: Summary Points

- A shockwave rate between 60 and 90 shocks per minute improves fragmentation.
- Routine ureteral stenting prior to shockwave lithotripsy is not indicated.
- Intravenous pyelogram or retrograde pyelogram can help localize poorly radiopaque stones during shockwave lithotripsy.
- Alpha-blockers improve stone free rates after shockwave lithotripsy and ureteroscopy.
- Confirm ureteral stone location with a retrograde pyelogram or semirigid ureteroscopy prior to placement of a ureteral access sheath during ureteroscopy.
- Always use a safety wire when performing ureteroscopy.
- Use a ureteral access sheath when multiple passes across the ureter are anticipated.
- Use smaller caliber instruments (baskets, lasers, etc.) through the flexible ureteroscope to preserve irrigation inflow and visualization as much as possible.
- If a stone basket cannot be disengaged from a basketed ureteral stone, disassemble the basket at the handle to allow removal of the ureteroscope.
- Balloon dilation of the distal ureter does not appear to increase ureteral stricture risk and can facilitate ureteral access for narrow ureteral orifices, reimplanted ureters and in men with large prostates.
- Most ureteroscopy complications can be safely managed by placing an indwelling ureteral stent for anywhere from 2 to 6 weeks.

References

1. Preminger GM, Tiselius HG, Assimos DG, et al. 2007 guideline for the management of ureteral calculi. Eur Urol. 2007;52:1610–31.
2. Semins MJ, Trock BJ, Matlaga BR. The effect of shock wave rate on the outcome of shock wave lithotripsy: a meta-analysis. J Urol. 2008;179:194–7.
3. Evan AP, McAteer JA, Connors BA, et al. Renal injury during shock wave lithotripsy is significantly reduced by slowing the rate of shock wave delivery. BJU Int. 2007;100:624–7.
4. Handa RK, McAteer JA, Connors BA, et al. Optimizing an escalating shockwave amplitude treatment strategy to protect the kidney from injury during shockwave lithotripsy. BJU Int. 2012;110:E1041–7.

5. Neucks JS, Pishchalnikov YA, Zancanaro AJ, et al. Improved acoustic coupling for shock wave lithotripsy. Urol Res. 2008;36:61–6.
6. Pishchalnikov YA, Neuks JS, VonDerHaar RJ, et al. Air pockets trapped during routine coupling in dry head lithotripsy can significantly decrease the delivery of shock wave energy. J Urol. 2006;176(6 pt 1):2706–10.
7. Sorensen MD, Bailey MR, Shah AR, et al. Quantitative assessment of shockwave lithotripsy accuracy and the effect of respiratory motion. J Endourol. 2012;26:1070–4.
8. Eichel L, Batzold P, Erturk E. Operator experience and adequate anesthesia improve treatment outcome with third-generation lithotripters. J Endourol. 2001;15:671–3.
9. Danuser H, Ackermann DK, Marth DC, et al. Extracorporeal shock wave lithotripsy in situ or after push-up for upper ureteral calculi: a prospective randomized trial. J Urol. 1993;150: 824–6.
10. Ghoneim IA, El-Ghoneimy MN, El-Naggar AE, et al. Extracorporeal shock wave lithotripsy in impacted upper ureteral stones: a prospective randomized comparison between stented and non-stented techniques. Urology. 2010;75:45–50.
11. Hara N, Koike H, Bilim V, et al. Efficiacy of extracorporeal shockwave lithotripsy with patients rotated supine or rotated prone for treating ureteral stones: a case-control study. J Endourol. 2006;20:170–4.
12. Zhu Y, Duijvesz D, Rovers MM, et al. Alpha-blockers to assist stone clearance after extracorporeal shock wave lithotripsy: a meta-analysis. BJU Int. 2010;106:256–61.
13. Schuler T, Shahani R, Honey RJ, et al. Medical expulsive therapy as an adjunct to improve shockwave lithotripsy outcomes: a systematic review and meta-analysis. J Endourol. 2009;23: 387–93.
14. Pittomvils G, Vandeursen H, Wevers M, et al. The influence of internal stone structure upon the fracture behaviour of urinary calculi. Ultrasound Med Biol. 1994;20:803–10.
15. Perks AE, Schuler TD, Lee J, et al. Stone attenuation and skin-to-stone distance on computed tomography predicts for stone fragmentation by shock wave lithotripsy. Urology. 2008;72: 765–9.
16. Nakada SY, Pearle MS, Soble JJ, et al. Extracoporeal shock-wave lithotripsy of middle ureteral stones: are ureteral stents necessary? Urology. 1995;46:649–52.
17. Pearle M, Nadler R, Bercowsky E, et al. Prospective randomized trial comparing shock wave lithotripsy and ureteroscopy for management of distal ureteral calculi. J Urol. 2001;166: 1255–60.
18. Thomas R, Cass AS. Extracorporeal shock wave lithotripsy in morbidly obese patients. J Urol. 1993;150:30–2.
19. Bach C, Nesar S, Kumar P, et al. The new digital flexible ureteroscopes: 'size does matter'—increased ureteric access sheath use! Urol Int. 2012;89:408–11.
20. Wallis MC, Brown DH, Jayanthi VR, et al. A novel technique for ureteral catheterization and/or retrograde ureteroscopy after cross-trigonal ureteral reimplantation. J Urol. 2003;170(4 Pt 2):1664–4.
21. Lezrek M, Ammani A, Bazine K, et al. The Split-leg modified lateral position for percutaneous renal surgery and optimal retrograde access to the upper urinary tract. Urology. 2011;78:217–20.
22. Zehri AA, Ather MH, Siddiqui KM, et al. A randomized clinical trial of lidocaine jelly for prevention of inadvertent retrograde stone migration during pneumatic lithotripsy of ureteral stone. J Urol. 2008;180:966–8.
23. Jeon SS, Hyun JH, Lee KS. A comparison of holmium: YAG laser with Lithoclast lithotripsy in ureteral calculi fragmentation. Int J Urol. 2005;12:544–7.
24. John TT, Razdan S. Adjunctive tamsulosin improves stone free rate after ureteroscopic lithotripsy of large renal and ureteric calculi: a prospective randomized study. Urology. 2010;75: 1040–2.
25. Dellis AE, Keeley Jr FX, Manolas V, et al. Role of alpha-blockers in the treatment of stent-related symptoms: a prospective randomized control study. Urology. 2014;83:56–61.

26. Bin X, Friedlander JL, Chuang KW, et al. Predictive factors for intraoperative balloon dilation in semirigid ureteroscopic lithotripsy. J Endourol. 2012;26:988–91.
27. El-Nahas AR, El-Tabey NA, Eraky I, et al. Semirigid ureteroscopy for ureteral stones: a multlivariate analysis of unfavorable results. J Urol. 2009;181:1158–62.
28. Massaro PA, Abdolell M, Norman RW. Assessing the accuracy of enoscopic estimates of lesion size in urology using in vitro models of the urinary tract. J Endourol. 2013;27: 1166–71.
29. Patel AP, Knudsen BE. Optimizing use of the holmium: YAG laser for surgical management or urinary lithiasis. Curr Urol Rep. 2014;15:397.

Chapter 13
Difficult Case: The Impacted Ureteral Stone

Sarah L. Coleman and Manoj Monga

The definition of an impacted ureteral stone was first described as the inability to pass a guide wire or catheter on initial attempts [1]. This definition has been criticized as the transient lie of the stone may explain failure to pass a guide wire. More recently, Mugiya at al. defined an impacted ureteral stone as a calculus causing ureteral obstruction and that remain in the same position for 2 months or greater [2]. A third definition cited in the literature is the failure to visualize contrast medium beyond the stone. All three definitions are used extensively in the literature and each in and of itself describe a challenging scenario for urologists. In our practice, an impacted stone is defined as an intraoperative finding. We consider an impacted stone as a stone where a guidewire will not pass without ancillary measures, which will be described in this chapter, and/or a stone that does not move when forceful irrigation is applied ureteroscopically.

Ureteral stone impaction is known to cause a local inflammatory response in the ureteral wall. Histologic examination of the ureter at the site of impacted stone will reveal chronic inflammation, interstitial fibrosis and urothelial hypertrophy which places these patients at risk for the development of ureteral strictures and ureteral polyps [2, 3]. Roberts et al. defined an impacted stone as a stone that had not changed location for at least 2 months, and reported a 24 % incidence of ureteral stricture with a mean follow-up of 7 months [4]. The main risk factor for stricture formation was ureteral peforation at the time of attempted stone removal. Ureteral strictures then place the patient at greater risk for future impacted stones as a result of the narrowed lumen. Chronic impaction is thought to cause local ischemia leading to fibrosis and edema [1]. It is thus essential that patients and physicians focus on preventing stone impaction to reduce the associated morbidity with treatment and long-term risk of ureteral stricture formation. Prevention of stone impaction requires treatment of stones prior to passage into the ureter or more ideally, prevention of stone formation in those identified to be at risk.

S.L. Coleman (✉) • M. Monga
Department of Endourology and Stone Disease, Stevan Streem Center,
Cleveland Clinic Foundation, Cleveland, OH, USA
e-mail: colemansarahlacy.coleman@gmail.com; mongam@ccf.org

S.R. Patel, S.Y. Nakada (eds.), *Ureteral Stone Management: A Practical Approach*, DOI 10.1007/978-3-319-08792-4_13

Stone size and stone location are major determining factors of the likelihood of spontaneous passage. The current AUA/EUA guidelines for ureteral calculi reported a spontaneous passage rate of 68 % (95 % CI: 48–85 %) for stones ≤5 mm and 47 % (95 % CI: 36–59 %) for stones >5 mm and ≤10 mm [5]. Multiple studies have supported the conclusion that the smaller the stone, the higher the likelihood of spontaneous passage. Impaction occurs when a stone traverses the ureter and the diameter of the stone exceeds the diameter of the ureteral lumen. The sites for impaction have classically been cited as the ureteropelvic junction, the crossing of the ureter over the iliac vessels and the ureterovesical junction. Recent literature suggests that the most common sites of impaction are the lower third of the ureter (53 %) and the upper third of the ureter (34 %) with the UPJ (3 %) and the site of crossing of the iliac vessels (3 %) less common than originally thought [6]. Treatment options are dependent on the location of stone impaction.

The best treatment modality for impacted ureteral stones is highly debated in the literature. Treatment options include extracorporeal shockwave lithotripsy (SWL), ureteroscopy (URS) and percutaneous approaches. Observation and medical expulsive therapy are also options that can be presented to the patient but they must be counseled on the risks of renal function deterioration, infection and pain.

Proximal impacted ureteral stones are amenable to all three treatment options. Distal impacted ureteral stones are best treated with retrograde ureteroscopy, though antegrade percutaneous ureteroscopy or laparoscopic ureterolithotomy may be considered for impacted distal ureteral stones >10 mm in size. SWL is an established treatment option for ureteral calculi but its efficacy in treating impacted ureteral stone has been questioned. The primary concern with SWL related to impacted ureteral stones relates to the expansion space theory [7]. This theory describes the lack of natural expansion space in the setting of an impacted stone. Additionally, stone impaction reduces the amount of water-stone interface essential to the effectiveness of SWL.

Multiple studies have compared the efficacy of SWL and URS for ureteral stones based on stone size, but few studies have examined the relative efficacy for these two modalities for impacted ureteral stones. Khalil et al. published a recent series of 37 patients treated with SWL and 45 patients treated with URS for impacted proximal ureteral stones and demonstrated statistically significant higher stone-free rates in URS group (80 %) compared to the SWL group (67.6 %) after one session [8]. The rate of ureteral perforation in this study was 6.7 %. Wu et al. published similar results in a series of patients with proximal ureteral stones. Stone impaction was not an inclusion criterion for this study but all patients had proximal ureteral stones >1 cm that failed to pass spontaneously [9]. Mugiya et al. performed retrograde URS on 104 patients with impacted stones and showed that the target stone was treated in all 104 patients with adjuvant SWL used in three cases all of whom had stones >3 cm. They conclude that URS should be first-line therapy for impacted ureteral stones [10]. Although more studies are needed to directly compare SWL and URS in the setting of stone impaction, the data available suggests that URS is superior to SWL in terms of stone-free rate and requirement for a second procedure.

SWL can be performed in an ambulatory setting without a general anesthetic and it is the least invasive, cheapest option. However, SWL has a lower success rate when compared to URS and more often requires a subsequent procedure. SWL additionally relies on the patient to pass residual stones fragments with the associated morbidity of flank pain, hematuria and steinstrasse. URS requires a general anesthetic and is more costly, but the stone-free rate is higher with fewer sessions required. Stent-related morbidity (hematuria, flank pain, voiding dysfunction and stent migration) is associated with retrograde ureteroscopic treatment of impacted stones. Ureteral perforation and stricture are complications unique to ureteroscopy but the risks are acceptably low. With the development of smaller caliber ureteroscopes and the introduction of the holmium: yttrium-aluminum-garnet (Ho:YAG) laser, ureteroscopy has become safer and more effective for the treatment of ureteral stones.

Percutaneous approaches to impacted ureteral calculi provide a third surgical option for management. The percutaneous nephrolithotomy technique allows for antegrade ureteroscopic management of impacted ureteral calculi. One main advantage to the percutaneous approach is access to renal calculi during the same procedure. Additionally, percutaneous access through a hydronephrotic renal pelvis spares the normal ureter distal to the stone. Often the ureter distal to an impacted stone will be edematous or tight; increasing the risk of perforation with a retrograde approach. In addition, an antegrade approach may allow extraction of the calculus without intracorporeal lithotripsy; decreasing the risk that stone fragments will become embedded in the edematous urothelium leading to stone granuloma and stricture. However, PCNL is associated with higher morbidity in the form of blood loss, pneumothorax, hemothorax, nephron damage, and damage to surrounding organs [11]. A recent randomized clinical trial of 174 patients with large (>15 mm) impacted proximal ureteral stones reported that outcomes were superior with an antegrade approach if the stone was located above the upper border of the fourth lumbar vertebra [12] (Fig. 13.1).

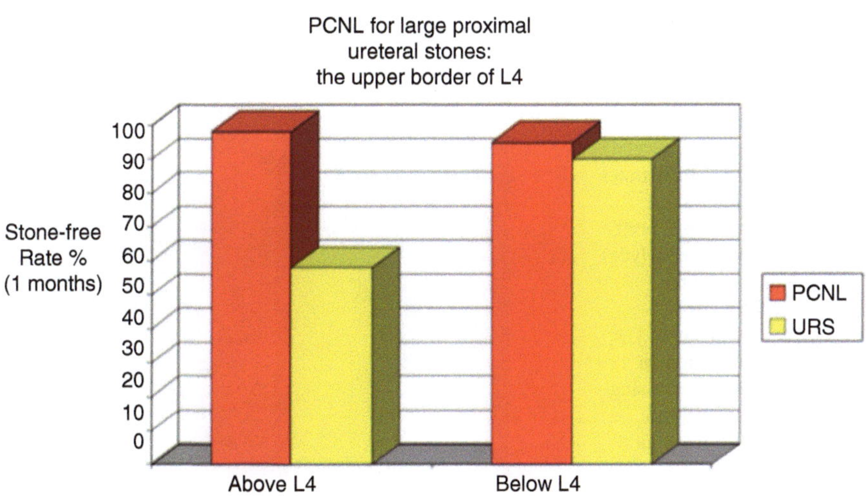

Fig. 13.1 Stone-free rates are superior with an antegrade percutaneous (PCNL) approach if the impacted proximal ureteral stone is above the level of L4 [12]

Case Report

A patient was referred after presenting with renal colic 3 months prior. She underwent ureteral stent placement followed by three sessions of extracorporeal shockwave lithotripsy. Prone KUB on referral to our center demonstrated significant residual stone burden in the proximal ureter and middle and lower calyces (Fig. 13.2). A CT scan was obtained due to concerns that the stent appeared to be lateral to the lie of the ureteral stone on KUB, raising the suspicion for either a perforation or a intramural stone fragment. CT scan confirmed that the proximal coil was outside of the collecting system and in addition thinning of the ureteral wall (Figs. 13.3 and 13.4). Due to parenchymal thinning on CT scan, a renal scan was obtained which

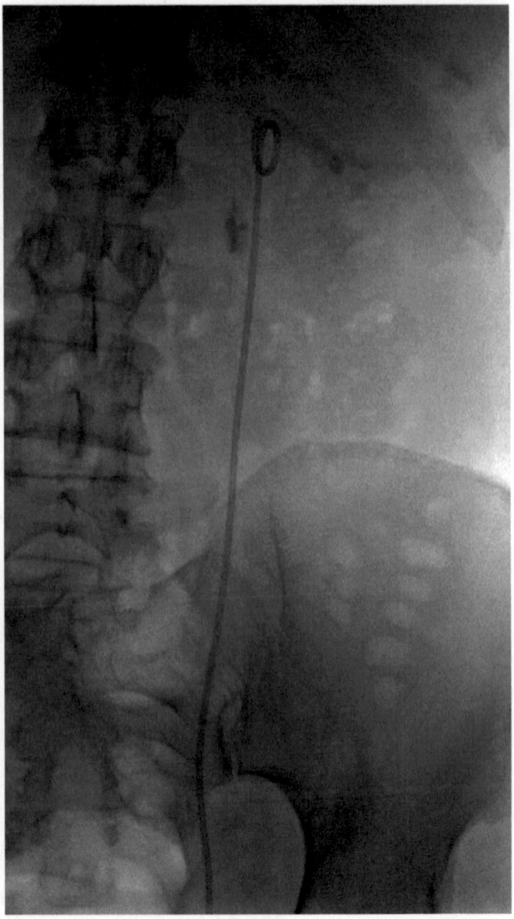

Fig. 13.2 KUB demonstrates significant residual stone burden in the proximal ureter and middle and lower calyces after stenting and three courses of SWL for an impacted ureteral stone. The stent appears to be too far lateral from the stone raising the suspicion for either a perforation or an intramural stone fragment

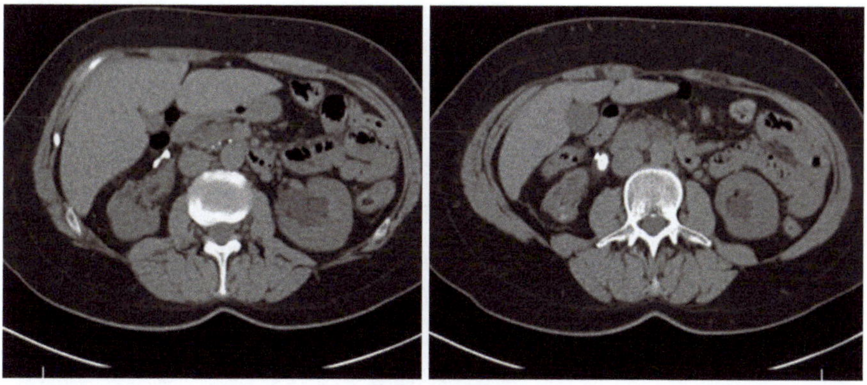

Fig. 13.3 CT scan confirmed that the proximal coil was outside of the collecting system

Fig. 13.4 Thinning of the ureteral wall associated with stone impaction

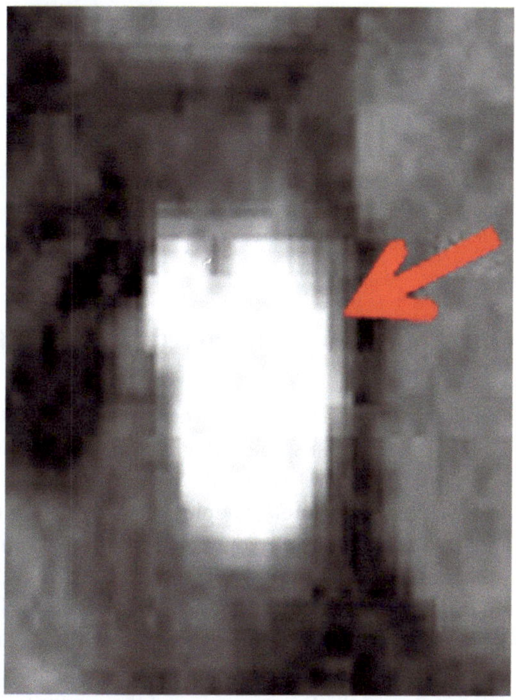

demonstrated 31 % split function on the affected side. A percutaneous antegrade approach was used to clear the impacted stone as well as the renal fragments, with removal of the misplaced ureteral stent (Fig. 13.5).

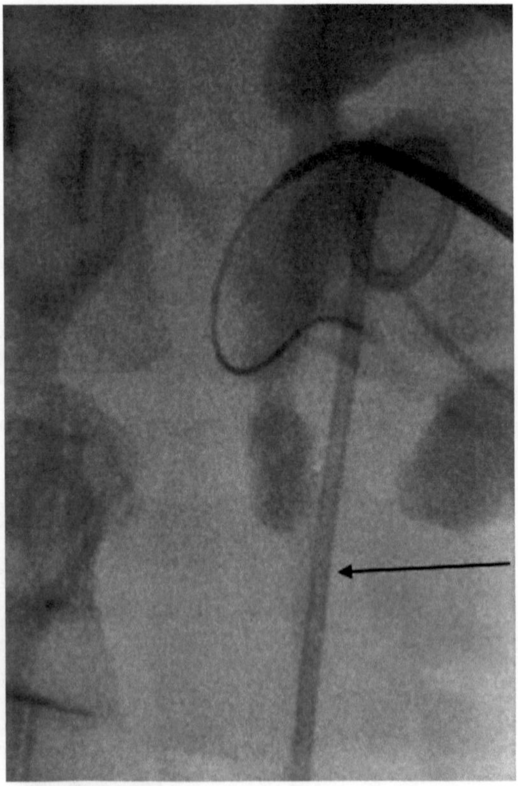

Fig. 13.5 A percutaneous antegrade approach was used to clear the impacted stone as well as the renal fragments, with removal of the misplaced ureteral stent

Our Approach to Impacted Ureteral Stones

Preoperative images are reviewed carefully. Duration of symptoms may be one factor that raises the suspicion that a stone may be impacted. On non-contrast CT, on occasion the ureteral wall will appear "thinned," raising concern for impaction, as will marked hydroureteronephrosis above the stone. If parenchymal thinning is noted, renal scintigraphy may be performed to quantify split renal function.

For stones <10 mm, a retrograde ureteroscopic approach is employed. Initial attempt is made to place a Sensor wire (Boston Scientific, Natick MA) cystoscopically past the point of obstruction. If the wire starts to buckle at the level of the stone, a 5-French open-ended catheter is advanced under fluoroscopic guidance to that point over the Sensor wire and the sensor wire is removed. A gentle retrograde pyelogram is performed to delineate the collecting system. A Glidewire (Terumo) is then advanced through the open-ended catheter and attempts to traverse the point of impaction are made. If the wire will not advance, it may be exchanged for an angled-glidewire. If this fails, 1–2 cc of lubricating jelly is gently instilled through the open-ended catheter and a final attempt at passage of the wire is made.

If the glidewire advances beyond the stone, the open-ended catheter is advanced over the glidewire to the ureteropelvic junction and the wire is removed. Contrast is instilled to confirm no perforation or submucosal false passage. The Sensor wire is then inserted for a more secure safety wire and the 5-Fr open-ended catheter is removed.

If the glidewire does not advance beyond the stone, then a semi-rigid ureteroscope (6Fr Tip) is advanced under direct vision to the level of the stone. A wire may be advanced under direct vision through the scope if a luminal opening is noted beside the stone. If no lumenal opening is identified, the stone can be carefully fragmented with the holmium laser until a lumen is created at which point the safety wire is inserted.

Once the wire is placed, the scope is removed and reinserted alongside the wire, with further fragmentation and clearance of the stone. In the face of an impacted stone, greater care is needed at all steps to avoid perforation. It is critical to clear all small fragments from the point of impaction before advancing the scope or a ureteral access sheath past this point – as failure to do so may lead to fragments embedding in the wall with subsequent stone granuloma and stricture. At times, the fragments may be too adherent to the inflamed mucosa, making extraction impossible (Fig. 13.6). If at any time during the retrograde ureteroscopic approach, the impacted stone cannot be clearly visualized or treated safely and there is no safety wire in place then a nephrostomy tube should be placed. The stone can then be treated via a percutaneous antegrade approach in the future or if an antegrade stent can be placed, a retrograde approach can be re-attempted once the stent has been allowed to passively dilate the ureter.

For stones >10 mm, we would recommend a percutaneous antegrade approach. A middle calyceal access will be optimal for access down the ureter with minimal morbidity, though an upper calyx may be selected if there are additional renal calculi to be addressed in the same setting. If the stone burden is limited to the ureter, a ureteral access sheath may be advanced down the ureter in lieu of tract dilation to 30Fr. As with a ureteroscopic approach, caution is necessary to avoid perforation, and if a guidewire does not advance easily past the point of impaction, it is

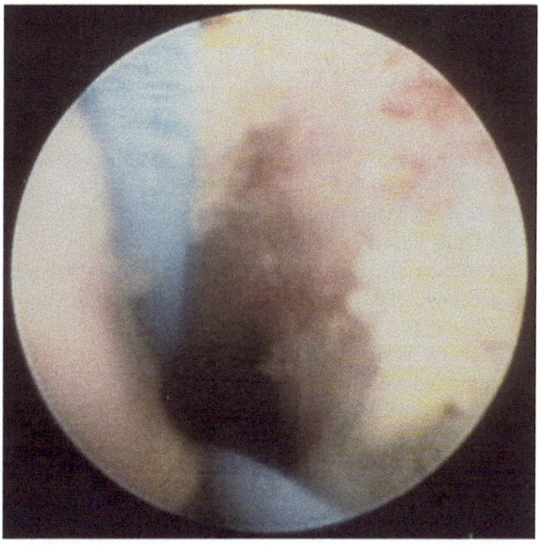

Fig. 13.6 Small fragments embedded in the edematous ureter at the completion of an antegrade ureteroscopy – risk factor for stricture formation

positioned above the stone and the sheath advanced to this point only. Laser fragmentation of the stone is performed, with forceful irrigation advancing fragments down to the bladder, and active basket extraction removing residual fragments. Once the site of impaction is cleared, the ureteroscope is advanced down to the bladder to evaluate for residual fragments.

After either a ureteroscopic or percutaneous approach for an impacted stone, a 7Fr Ureteral stent is left for 2 weeks. A tubeless approach is used for all antegrade procedures. Though we typically utilize selective imaging after endoscopic procedures, an impacted stone would be one of the important criteria where routine imaging is performed; in our series 27 % of patients with an impacted stone developed a stricture on follow-up [13]. A diuretic renal scan is performed 4 weeks after stent removal, and if normal, is repeated at 3 months, 6 months and 1 year. If delayed drainage is noted on follow-up, a retrograde pyelogram is performed to delineate the site and length of stricture; and will typically be addressed by a reconstructive procedure, dictated by these intraoperative findings.

Take Home Messages

- We recommend an antegrade ureteroscopic approach for impacted ureteral stones >10 mm and a retrograde ureteroscopic approach for impacted ureteral stones <10 mm.
- There is a limited role for SWL for impacted ureteral stones.
- Caution should be exercised during the treatment of impacted ureteral stones as they are at a high risk for perforation and can predispose to ureteral stricture.
- Renal scan should be performed to evaluate renal function if significant thinning of renal parenchyma is noted on CT scan.

References

1. Morgentaler A, Bridge SS, Dretler SP. Management of the impacted ureteral calculus. J Urol. 1990;143:263–6.
2. Mugiya S, Maruyama S, Hadano S, Nagae H. Endoscopic features of impacted ureteral stones. J Urol. 2004;171:89–91.
3. Huffman JL, Bagley DH, Lyon ES. Abnormal ureter and intrarenal collecting system. In: Urologic endoscopy: a manual and atlas. Boston: Little Brown and Co.; 1985. p. 59–73. Chapter 6.
4. Roberts WW, Cadeddu JA, Micali S, et al. Ureteral stricture formation after removal of impacted calculi. J Urol. 1998;159:723–6.
5. Preminger GM, Tiselius HG, Assimos DF, et al. 2007 Guideline for the management of ureteral calculi. J Urol. 2007;178:2418–34.
6. El-Barky E, Ali Y, Sahsah M, et al. Site of impaction of ureteric calculi requiring surgical intervention. Urolithiasis. 2014;42:67–73.

7. Chaussy CG, Fuchs GJ. Current state and future developments of noninvasive treatment of human urinary stones with extracorporeal shock wave lithotripsy. J Urol. 1989;141: 782–9.
8. Khalil M. Management of impacted proximal ureteral stone: extracorporeal shock wave lithotripsy versus ureteroscopy with holmium: YAG laser lithotripsy. Urol Ann. 2013;5: 88–92.
9. Wu CF, Shee JJ, Lin WY, et al. Comparison between extracorporeal shock wave lithotripsy and semirigid ureterorenoscope with holmium:YAG laser lithotripsy for treating large proximal ureteral stones. J Urol. 2004;172:1899–902.
10. Mugiya S, Nagato M, Un-No T, et al. Endoscopic management of impacted ureteral stones using a small caliber ureteroscope and a laser lithotripter. J Urol. 2000;164:329–31.
11. Maheshwari PN, Oswal AT, Andankar M, et al. Is antegrade ureteroscopy better than retrograde ureteroscopy for impacted large upper ureteral calculi? J Endourol. 1999;13:441–4.
12. Li H, Na W, Li H, et al. Percutaneous nephrolithotomy versus ureteroscopic lithotomy for large (>15 mm) impacted upper ureteral stones in different locations: is the upper border of the fourth lumbar vertebra a good indication for choice of management method? J Endourol. 2013;27:1120–5.
13. Adiyat KT, Meuleners R, Monga M. Selective postoperative imaging after ureteroscopy. Urology. 2009;73:490–3.

Chapter 14
Difficult Case: Ureteral Stricture Distal to a Stone

Necole M. Streeper and Stephen Y. Nakada

Introduction

Ureteral stricture is a late complication of ureteroscopy (URS) and can be challenging to treat stones when present concomitantly. Ureteral stones may fail to spontaneously pass secondary to a distally located ureteral stricture. Retrograde access may be difficult or unable to be obtained depending on the degree of the stricture and presence of stone impaction. This chapter will focus on the treatment options for a ureteral stone with a distal ureteral stricture (Fig. 14.1).

Pre-operative Considerations

Patients with a history of difficult or impacted stones, multiple prior ureteroscopies, abdominal surgeries or radiation therapy are prone to ureteral stricture formation. A detailed history of prior stone events and surgical intervention should be obtained, including prior surgical complications. Pre-operative imaging with a non-contrast computed tomography (CT) scan may not suggest presence of a ureteral stricture in the setting of a ureteral stone. Urinary tract infections should be treated with antibiotics prior to any surgical intervention. It is also important to discuss with the patient realistic expectations of the surgery with the possibility of multiple procedures when the presence of a ureteral stricture and/or impacted stone is suspected.

N.M. Streeper (✉) • S.Y. Nakada
Department of Urology, University of Wisconsin School of Medicine and Public Health, Madison, WI, USA
e-mail: streeper@urology.wisc.edu; nakada@urology.wisc.edu

S.R. Patel, S.Y. Nakada (eds.), *Ureteral Stone Management: A Practical Approach*, DOI 10.1007/978-3-319-08792-4_14

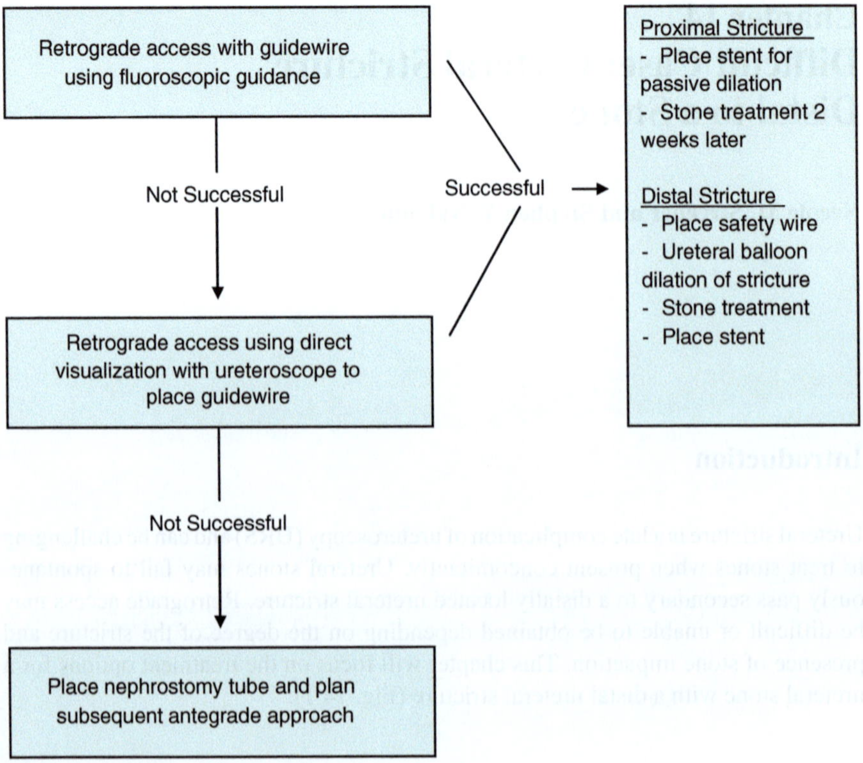

Fig. 14.1 Treatment of a ureteral stone with distal ureteral stricture

Retrograde vs Antegrade Ureteral Access

In the setting of a concomitant ureteral stricture and stone, it may be difficult to gain retrograde access. Often times the stone is impacted at the location of the ureteral stricture making access even more challenging. An attempt should be made to pass a guidewire, such as the Sensor (Boston Scientific, Natick, MA, USA), under fluoroscopic visualization. If there is difficulty bypassing the stone a 5F ureteral access catheter should be passed under fluoroscopic guidance over the guidewire to a position just distal to the obstruction. The wire should be removed in order to perform a retrograde pyelogram (RPG) to delineate the anatomy. The ureteral access catheter will also straighten out the ureter distal to the obstruction allowing for the guidewire to project in a more favorable orientation. Using the imaging gained from the RPG a hydrophilic guidewire, such as a glidewire, should then be re-advanced through the ureteral access catheter to negotiate past the obstructing segment. It is important to carefully manipulate the guidewire with care in order to avoid ureteral perforation. Glidewires are often able to bypass an impacted stone or obstructing stricture and are less likely to cause a false passage or ureteral perforation. There are both straight and angled glidewires available. Once the glidewire is coiled within the renal pelvis, the ureteral access catheter should be passed over the wire and above the area of obstruction. If the urine draining from the access catheter appears to be infected then the procedure should be abandoned, a stent should be placed and treatment should be performed after appropriate antibiotics have eradicated the infection. Otherwise, the glidewire should then be exchanged for a stiffer guidewire to avoid the glidewire from inadvertently being removed.

If the above maneuver is not successful then the next step is placement of the guidewire under direct visualization. A guidewire should be left in place just below the area of obstruction and the ureteroscope, either semi-rigid if within the distal ureter or flexible if within the mid/proximal ureter, should be passed to the level of the obstruction. Under direct visualization the diameter of the stricture, size of the stone, and presence of stone impaction may be assessed. The guidewire may then be directed around the stricture and stone at a favorable appearing location. If stone impaction prevents this, then laser lithotripsy may be carefully performed until a guidewire is able to be passed. It is not recommended to attempt basketing the stone without a safety wire in place. In cases of failed retrograde access a percutaneous nephrostomy tube should be placed with plans for antegrade ureteroscopy.

Percutaneous antegrade treatment of ureteral stones is a secondary treatment after failed retrograde access to the stone. A stone positioned in the ureter just proximal to a ureteral stricture may be best approached in this manner before a standard endoureterotomy is performed. An upper-posterior or mid-posterior caliceal approach to percutaneous access offers the most direct route to the ureter. Flexible antegrade URS with laser lithotripsy may then be performed. A nephrostomy tube should be replaced to perform an antegrade nephrostogram postoperatively to evaluate the location and extent of the ureteral stricture for definitive surgical treatment.

After successful retrograde access the next step is determined by the location of the stricture that is compromising access to the stone. Due to the fragility of the proximal ureter, it is best to stent and allow for passive dilation rather than active dilation with a ureteral balloon dilator. A second-look URS may be done in 1–2 weeks, typically with an easily accessible ureter. Passive dilation is a safe and effective way to dilate the ureter; however, it does require two separate procedures. For distal ureteral strictures, a safety wire should be placed prior to balloon dilation. The safety wire may be placed with a dual lumen catheter, 8/10 dilator, ureteral access sheath, or under direct visualization with the semi-rigid ureteroscope.

Ureteral Balloon Dilation

Ureteral balloon dilators are recommended for dilation of ureteral strictures that compromise access to the ureteral stone. Use of balloon dilators are associated with increased post-operative pain and should only be used when necessary [1]. Balloon

Table 14.1 Specifications of current ureteral balloon dilators

Balloon Dilator	Inflated Balloon Diameter (mm)	Balloon Length (cm)	Rated Burst Pressure (atm)
Cook			
Ascend AQ	12Fr, 15Fr, 18Fr, 21Fr, or 30Fr	4, 6, or 10 cm	20
Boston Scientific			
UroMax Ultra	12Fr, 15Fr, 18Fr, 21Fr, 24Fr, or 30Fr	4, 6, 8 or 10 cm	20
Bard			
UroForce	12Fr, 15Fr, 18Fr, 21Fr or 24Fr	4, 6 of 10 cm	23

dilators range in length from 4 to 10 cm with various diameters, 12–15F, see Table 14.1 for specifications. The balloon has radiopaque markers at the proximal and distal ends, which are used to position the balloon over the working guidewire using fluoroscopy (Fig. 14.2). They should never be inflated over an obstructing ureteral stone due to the risk of ureteral perforation. Once the balloon is in proper position, it is inflated with half-strength contrast using a pressure gauge syringe. The balloons typically can withstand inflation pressures up to 17–20 atm; however dilation of the ureter typically can be achieved at lower pressures (4–6 atm). The lowest pressure necessary to dilate the ureter should be used to avoid ureteral perforation, and therefore it is important to inflate the balloon under fluoroscopic guidance. Typically a "waist" is seen in the balloon at the location of the stricture, and one should continue to inflate slowly until the "waist" disappears. The balloon is then deflated and removed, leaving the guidewire in place. Ureteroscopy may then be performed to treat the stone. Complications that can occur with balloon dilation include: balloon rupture from over inflation, mucosal injury, bleeding, and ureteral perforation if inflation is performed too rapidly or if higher pressures are used than necessary.

Post-operative Imaging

Patients should be monitored with post-operative imaging to evaluate for possible recurrent asymptomatic ureteral strictures. We routinely perform renal ultrasound 4 weeks after stent removal to evaluate for hydronephrosis. If hydronephrosis is present, evaluation should include RPG, intravenous pyelogram (IVP) or delayed contrast CT imaging. If no hydronephrosis is present, repeat renal ultrasound at 6–12 months post-operatively should be done to assess for late ureteral stricture

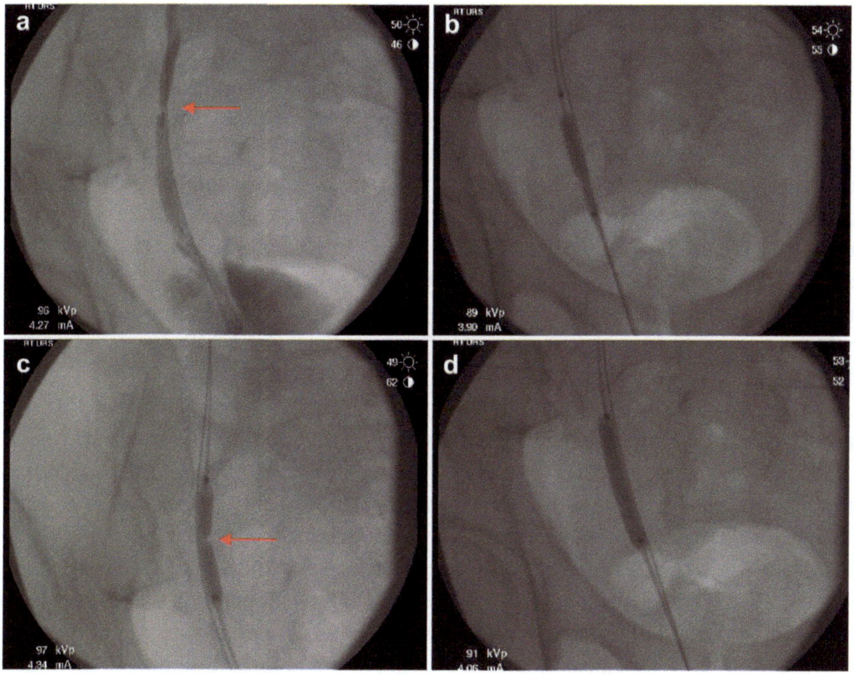

Fig. 14.2 Balloon dilation of a ureteral stricture. (**a**) A retrograde pyelogram (RPG) is performed to evaluate the area of obstruction. The *arrow* indicates the location of the ureteral stricture. (**b**) The balloon has radiopaque markers at the proximal and distal ends, which is used to position the balloon over the working guidewire using fluoroscopy. Once the balloon is in proper position, it is inflated with half-strength contrast using a pressure gauge syringe. (**c**) It is important to inflate the balloon under fluoroscopic guidance to dilate the stricture with the lowest pressure required. Typically a "waist" is seen in the balloon at the location of the stricture as indicated by the *arrow*. (**d**) The balloon is inflated slowly until the "waist" disappears

formation. It is possible to have silent obstruction and if routine imaging is not done to evaluate the patient may risk loss of the renal unit. Weizer et al. found a 3.7 % ureteral obstruction rate after ureteroscopy in asymptomatic patients within 3 months post-operatively suggesting a need for routine imaging [2]. Adiyat et al. found an overall ureteral stricture rate of 1.4 % after ureteroscopy with all cases involving stone impaction, balloon dilation, or ureteral perforation suggesting that routine imaging may not be necessary after uncomplicated ureteroscopy [3].

Complications and Ureteral Stricture Formation

Ureteral false passage is a complication that can occur with attempted passage of a guidewire across a strictured ureter or impacted stone [4]. The ureteral wall mucosa is perforated in this type of injury, but the wall itself remains intact. Recognition of the injury is the first step, followed by correct placement of the guidewire with confirmation by RPG. A ureteral stent should then be placed to allow the false passage to heal for 2 weeks. False passage is associated with a post-operative ureteral stricture rate of 0.4–0.9 %, despite intra-operative recognition [5].

The risk of ureteral perforation is increased in cases of impacted stones or ureteral strictures with difficult ureteral access. It may occur with the advancement of guidewires, ureteroscopes or aggressive ureteral balloon dilation. Treatment of a ureteral perforation typically involves termination of the procedure and placement of a ureteral stent. The stent should be left in place for 4–6 weeks prior to the second procedure. Taie et al. found a ureteral perforation rate of 1.2 % in a large review of patients undergoing ureteroscopy [6]. However, they did not evaluate the rate in complicated cases. Longer operative times have also been associated with an increased rate of ureteral perforation [7].

Ureteral strictures are a late complication of ureteroscopy that can lead to loss of renal function. Recent studies suggest that the overall incidence of ureteral stricture after ureteroscopy is 0.5–3.5 % [8–10]. The cause of ureteral strictures is multifactorial; primarily due to trauma during ureteroscopy from mechanical or thermal injury. Impacted stones may cause severe inflammation and vascular compromise that leads to stricture formation. Roberts et al. found that the rate of ureteral stricture disease after URS of impacted calculi was 24 %, much higher than the less than 1 % noted in the general population of calculi treated with ureteroscopy [11]. Ureteral perforation is another cause of stricture formation secondary to injury to the ureter. Stoller et al. found a ureteral stricture rate of 5.9 % in patients with intraoperative ureteral perforation, compared to an overall 3.5 % rate [8].

Treatment of Ureteral Strictures

Ureteral strictures should not be treated with endoureterotomy at the same time as stone treatment because of potential for fragments to migrate into the periureteral space secondary to ureteral perforation. The current management of ureteral strictures depends on the length and location. Short, non-ischemic, ureteral strictures <2 cm in length generally have good results from an endoscopic approach. Strictures that are >2 cm or ischemic are better managed with open/laparoscopic/robotic-assisted approaches that include ureteroureterostomy, Boari flap, psoas hitch, ileal ureter or auto transplantation depending on the length and location. Initial treatment involves obtaining imaging with combined retrograde and antegrade pyelogram to visualize the length of the stricture in order to plan the appropriate operative approach. CT urogram may be indicated if extrinsic or malignant causes of stricture formation are suspected as it will provide additional anatomic information. If diminished renal function is suspected then renal scintigraphy with diuretic washout should be performed to ensure the kidney has adequate function prior to stricture repair. This should be performed after the system is adequately drained with a ureteral stent or nephrostomy tube in order to optimize renal function.

Endoscopic management of ureteral strictures may be accomplished with a holmium laser incision, cold knife incision or balloon dilation in a retrograde or antegrade fashion. Incision provides better results than balloon dilation. Overall success rates for endoscopic treatment of benign ureteral strictures is approximately 80–85 % [12, 13]. The density, length and cause of the stricture may affect the success rate. After treatment a ureteral stent should be left in place for approximately 3–6 weeks, and follow-up imaging after removal of the stent is necessary to evaluate long-term success. Post-operative imaging may include: renal ultrasound, excretory urography, retrograde pyelogram, or renal scintigraphy with diuretic washout. Renal ultrasound is the preferred imaging because it is well-tolerated and adequately evaluates for the presence of hydronephrosis. Typically this is performed 3 months post-operatively and on a yearly basis if the patient remains asymptomatic. If there is hydronephrosis or thinning of the renal parenchyma on ultrasound, this may be further evaluated with contrasted studies or renal scintigraphy.

Take Home Points

- Balloon dilators are never inflated over an obstructing ureteral stone because of the risk of ureteral perforation.
- Ureteral strictures should not be treated with endoureterotomy at the same time as stone treatment because of the potential for fragments to migrate into the periureteral space secondary to ureteral perforation.
- If unable to obtain retrograde ureteral access, then a nephrostomy tube should be placed with plans for antegrade ureteroscopic approach.
- Evaluate for asymptomatic obstruction post-operatively with imaging after ureteral stent removal.

References

1. Kourambas J, Byrne RR, Preminger GM. Does a ureteral access sheath facilitate ureteroscopy? J Urol. 2001;165(3):789–93.
2. Weizer AZ, Auge BK, Silverstein AD, Delvecchio FC, Brizuela RM, Dahm P, et al. Routine postoperative imaging is important after ureteroscopic stone manipulation. J Urol. 2002; 168(1):46–50.
3. Adiyat KT, Meuleners R, Monga M. Selective postoperative imaging after ureteroscopy. Urol J. 2009;73(3):490–3.
4. Kau EL, Ng CS, Fuchs GJ. Complications of ureteroscopic surgery. In: Taneja SS, editor. Complications of urologic surgery. 4th ed. Philadelphia: Elsevier; 2010. p. 303–16.
5. Johnson DB, Pearle MS. Complications of ureteroscopy. Urol Clin North Am. 2004;31(1): 157–71.
6. Taie K, Jasemi M, Khazaeli D, Fatholahi A. Prevalence and management of complications of ureteroscopy: a seven-year experience with introduction of a new maneuver to prevent ureteral avulsion. Urol J. 2012;9(1):356–60.

7. Schuster TG, Hollenbeck BK, Faerber GJ, Wolf Jr JS. Complications of ureteroscopy: analysis of predictive factors. J Urol. 2001;166(2):538–40.
8. Stoller ML, Wolf Jr JS, Hofmann R, Marc B. Ureteroscopy without routine balloon dilation: an outcome assessment. J Urol. 1992;147(5):1238–42.
9. Delvecchio FC, Auge BK, Brizuela RM, Weizer AZ, Silverstein AD, Lallas CD, et al. Assessment of stricture formation with the ureteral access sheath. Urology. 2003;61(3):518–22.
10. Harmon WJ, Sershon PD, Blute ML, Patterson DE, Segura JW. Ureteroscopy: current practice and long-term complications. J Urol. 1997;157(1):28–32.
11. Roberts WW, Cadeddu JA, Micali S, Kavoussi LR, Moore RG. Ureteral stricture formation after removal of impacted calculi. J Urol. 1998;159:723–6.
12. Wolf Jr JS, Elashry OM, Clayman RV. Long-term results of endoureterotomy for benign ureteral and ureteroenteric strictures. J Urol. 1997;158(3):759–64.
13. Corcoran AT, Smaldone MC, Ricchiuti DD, Averch TD. Management of benign ureteral strictures in the endoscopic era. J Endourol. 2009;23(11):1909–12.

Chapter 15
Complications in the Treatment of Ureteral Stones: Prevention and Management

Stavros Sfoungaristos and Mordechai Duvdevani

Introduction

Medical technology progress, increased surgical experience and smaller diameter instruments have contributed in making ureteroscopy a safe and widely utilized procedure for the management of ureteral stones. Although the complications rate is low, some complications can be very dangerous for the patient. The present chapter will focus on the most common complications during ureteroscopic stone procedures, analyze the causative factors and suggest tips to avoid and manage them.

Ureteral Bleeding

Intraoperative bleeding represents a rare complication of ureteroscopy and it rarely represents the cause of termination of the procedure due to compromised visualization of the ureteral lumen. Causes of bleeding include trauma of the ureteral orifice during the insertion of the ureteroscope, pelvis or caliceal over-distension, mucosal injury during insertion of stiff guidewires or stone manipulation with basket.

Tepeler et al. reported and categorized the intraoperative complications in 1,208 patients who underwent ureteroscopy for stone removal [1]. The authors reported that the incidence of intraoperative bleeding was 1.9 % and none of the cases needed

S. Sfoungaristos
Department of Urology, Hadassah Hebrew University Medical Center, Jerusalem, Israel
e-mail: sfoungaristosst@gmail.com

M. Duvdevani (✉)
Department of Urology, Hadassah Ein-Kerem University Hospital,
The Hebrew University, Jerusalem, Israel
e-mail: moti_duv@yahoo.com

S.R. Patel, S.Y. Nakada (eds.), *Ureteral Stone Management: A Practical Approach*, DOI 10.1007/978-3-319-08792-4_15

blood transfusion. Although bleeding was minor in most of the cases, four of them (0.33 %) were terminated due to loss of vision.

Geavlete et al. retrospectively reviewed 2,735 ureteroscopic procedures operated in a single center between 1994 and 2005 [2]. The incidence of significant bleeding during the ureteroscopic procedure was 0.1 % with three of the cases having to be terminated due to limited visualization. All cases were managed with stent placement and no blood transfusion was required.

Toepfer et al. compared the clinical outcome of rigid ureteroscopy between patients who receive antiplatelet and anticoagulant therapy and patients who did not [3]. They reported no differences in bleeding complications. Similarly, Watterson et al. reviewed 29 stones of patients with known bleeding diathesis who were treated with holmium laser intracorporeal lithotripsy [4]. All procedures were finished uneventfully, apart from one case in which a blood transfusion was required due to a significant retroperitoneal hemorrhage. Of great interest, in this specific patient he was treated with laser and concomitant electrohydraulic lithotripsy (which has a higher rate of ureteral perforation and ureteal damage compared to the Holmium laser).

In the contemporary era, smaller diameter ureteroscopes have decreased the need for ureteral orifice dilation and thereby the incidence of significant bleeding [5]. The surgeon may also decrease the risk of intraoperative bleeding by decreasing the use of extraction tools, like baskets, and stiff wires. A flexible instrument should be used in cases that there is an increased resistance to pass proximal the ureter. Whenever, the visualization is low and manipulations inside the ureter are not safe, a ureteral stent should be placed and the procedure should be terminated. Bleeding is then generally controlled within a few hours. In the rare case of uncontrolled bleeding, a tamponade balloon catheter may be used intraoperatively. Persistent, life-threatening hemorrhage should be managed with immediate angioembolization.

Ureteral Wall Thermal Injury

Some of the devices used for intracorporeal lithotripsy, mainly electrohydraulic and laser lithotripters, produce thermal energy during stone fragmentation. As a result of the above phenomenon, thermal injury of the ureteral wall, even if it is rare, represents a potential complication of the procedure. Direct contact of the electrohydraulic probe to the ureteral wall may lead to ureteral perforation due to coagulative necrosis. The same results can be produced by the Holmium laser fiber which has a penetration depth of 0.5 mm. However, when the tip is located adistance of at least 2 mm away from the ureteral wall, the possibilities of thermal injury are rare.

Sofer et al. reported a thermal injury incidence of 0.2 % in 598 patients who were treated with Holmium laser lithotripsy [6]. On the other hand, this rate was significantly higher (1 %) in a series of 198 patients who were managed with electrohydraulic lithotripsy by Basar et al. [7].

In depth knowledge of the technical characteristics of ureteroscopic instruments, surgical experience and appropriate instrumentation during lithotripsy are the mainstays for decreasing the potential of ureteral wall thermal injury. In cases of ureteral wall injury or ureteral perforation, a stent should be placed to allow for mucosal healing. Future CT urography may be helpful for early identification of ureteral stricture and obstruction.

Ureteral Abrasion

Mucosal abrasion represents the most common complication of ureteroscopic procedures. There is no standardized definition and it is rarely of clinical significance apart from technical difficulties that can be produced during the operation mainly due to obstruction of the lumen and decrease of visibility. It is obvious that any instrument that passes through the ureter can produce a certain degree of abrasion. This degree is higher when rigid and semirigid instruments are used, and multiple entries of the ureteroscope are needed for stone disintegration and removal. Butler et al. reported a 0.3 % rate of mucosal abrasion in a study of 2,273 ureteroscopies. They reported that the ureteroscope itself was the cause of mucosal abrasion in all cases [8]. Similarly, Geavlete et al. reported that mucosal abrasion was noticed in 1.5 % of 2,735 ureteroscopic procedures made with semirigid instruments of variable diameter ranged from 6.5 to 10F [2].

The flexibility and size of the ureteroscope can be correlated to the degree of mucosal abrasion [9]. Francesca et al. thus compared the safety of conventional rigid ureteroscopes with a diameter from 9.5 to 11.5Fr and semirigid ureteroscope with a diameter ranging between 6 and 7Fr [9]. Ureteral mucosal abrasion was observed in 24 % of 248 rigid ureteroscopies and in 6 % of 49 semirigid procedures. The authors conclude that small caliber semirigid ureteroscopes are safer compared to conventional instruments.

Theoretically, small abrasions will not affect the procedure in terms of technical aspects and clinical outcome. They usually do not need any adjuvant procedure since they will heal fast without long term complications.

Creation of a False Passage

False passage represents a common complication during endoscopic maneuvers. The reported rate is widely varied and ranges from 1 to 18.3 % [2, 10]. Although it is characterized as a minor complication, it can be transformed into a serious complication if it is not identified and left untreated. It is generally caused during the insertion of a guidewire and it is more common to happen at sites of ureteral inflammation or impacted stones. Ureteral strictures, tight ureteral orifice, tortuous ureters and excessive force during the insertion of the ureteroscope may also lead to false passage. Blind manipulations of any endoscopic equipment, such as baskets, laser fibers and forceps may lead to creation of false passage, as well.

Suspicious clinical signs such as difficulty in advancing the wire through the ureter should be carefully noted and if the manipulation is continued may lead to a false passage. The fluoroscopic identification of the wire inside the pelvis and the caliceal system does not exclude the presence of a false passage, since the wire may re-enter the ureteral lumen after a short sub-mucosal course. The latter situation may lead to tract dilatation with a ureteral catheter or with the ureteroscope. Dilatation of a false passage with a balloon can lead to disaster as it can then lead to ureteral perforation and increased ureteral damage.

In case that a false passage is suspected, then a dual-lumen catheter can be inserted and a retrograde ureterography is performed. The absence of contrast material within the pelvis or the presence of contrast collection along the ureteral wall in both images would confirm the findings of a false passage or of ureteral perforation. In case that this is confirmed, the wire should be removed and replaced. Ideally, wire removal and re-insertion should be performed under vision with the ureteroscope just distally to the submucosal root. If the false root is very long, a double J stent should be left and the procedure should be repeated after 2 weeks.

Ureteral Perforation

Perforation of the ureter represents a common complications of ureteroscopy. The rate of this complication was significantly higher in the first steps of minimal invasive surgery of the ureter as a result of epidural anesthesia, larger instruments and minimal experience.

The introduction of smaller diameters ureteroscopes dramatically changed the perforation rates during ureteroscopy. Abdel-Razzak and Bagley reported 1 case of perforation out of 65 patients treated with a 6.9F semirigid ureteroscope [5]. The same authors found 1.7 % perforation rate in 290 procedures performed by flexible ureteroscopes with tip diameter ranging from 8.5 to 10F [11]. To provide the significance of instrument diameter on ureteral perforation rates, Grasso and Bagley described their experience with flexible ureteroscopes smaller than 8F [12]. No ureteral perforation was observed in 584 ureteroscopic procedures.

Apart from instrument diameter, the lithotripter unit/laser fiber itself may perforate the ureter. Many different kinds of available instruments (laser fibers, guidewires, stone extraction baskets) can produce such a complication. This can be the result either of a bad operator maneuver either from direct contact of the tip of the lithotripter (laser fiber or EHL tip) with the ureteral epithelium. The evolution in Holmium laser fibers has contributed in increased safety due to technical aspects. The penetration depth of contemporary laser fibers has been described to be approximately 0.5 mm and thus it can be used in very close distance to the ureteral wall without damaging the adjacent organs. The above is mainly useful when we treat urothelial tumors by laser ablation.

As we described above, electrohydraulic lithotripter (EHL) may perforate the ureteral wall due to coagulative necrosis following direct contact with the mucosa.

Billen et al. reported that electrohydraulic lithotripter may be associated with higher rates of complications [13]. In their study they observed 4 cases of perforation out of 13 patients treated with ureteroscopy and intracorporeal lithotripsy.

Sozen et al. described their experience of 500 patients with ureteral calculi managed with ureteroscopy and pneumatic lithotripter with Swiss lithoclast [14]. Ureteral perforation was observed in 1.4 % of the patients. The same year, Aghamir et al. reported their results of 340 patients and 362 ureteral calculi treated with a 8.5F ureteroscope and Swiss lithoclast [15]. The rate of ureteral perforation was 0.27 % providing the safety of pneumatic lithotripter.

The efficacy and safety of the two above lithotripters, pneumatic and electrohydraulic, were compared in a randomized, prospective study by Hofbauer et al. The authors studied 72 patients with ureteral calculi. Interestingly, they found that perforation rates were significantly higher in favor of pneumatic lithotripter (17.6 % versus 2.6 % for electrohydraulic and pneumatic lithotripter, respectively) [16].

More recently, Sun et al. compared the safety of the Swiss lithoclast pneumatic lithotripter and Holmium: YAG laser for the treatment of 285 consecutive patients with ureteral stones [17]. No perforations were observed in the group managed with laser lithotripsy. In contrast, they found five cases with ureteral perforation in the group of pneumatic lithotripter. Similar results were reported by Sofer et al. as the authors observed only a single perforation case out of 598 patients who were treated by Holmium: YAG lithotripsy [6].

The above observations guide us to conclude that laser lithotripsy should be considered the modality of choice as it can provide increased safety during ureteroscopic lithotripsy.

Apart from ureteroscopes and lithotripters, any unit that is used during the procedure and that enters the ureteral lumen may potentially perforate the organ. Such equipments include baskets, guidewires, ureteral dilatators, and ureteral catheters. Although perforation can be managed efficiently by stent placement without major long-term complications, it can be dangerous if not recognized during the procedure and left untreated. This may happen more commonly when we insert instruments, like wires or ureteral catheters, without direct vision. Thus, ureteral consistency should be always checked at the end of the procedure in order to identify a ureteral perforation early and thus appropriately manage it. Increased intra-pelviceal or intra-calyceal pressures may result in ureteral perforation, often wider than the ones produced by instruments. This can occur in cases where high pressure irrigation is used for intra-ureteral fluid flow. The transmission of high pressures into the collecting system may lead to rupture of the ureteral or pelvic wall, especially in renal units with small non-dilated collecting systems and an intra-renal pelvis.

The majority of perforations are small and can be managed conservatively. In all cases, a safety guide wire should be in place because otherwise the insertion of a wire through a ruptured ureter can even enlarge the rupture site transforming a minor complication into a major one. Over the wire, a double J stent can be inserted and left in place for 4–6 weeks. CT urography is advised for early identification of a ureteral stricture at the perforation site. In cases of large, longitudinal perforations that cannot be managed conservatively, open or laparoscopic repair may be the treatment of choice.

Ureteral Avulsion

Ureteral avulsion represents the most dramatic complication that can be encountered during ureteroscopic procedures. It may occur in cases that forceful insertion of the ureteroscope is attempted or large stone fragments are manipulated within a smaller diameter lumen. The proximal part of the ureter is at a greater risk for avulsion due to less muscle support compared to the distal ureter.

The use of multiple wire baskets has been implicated as a causative factor for ureteral avulsion. The newer nitinol tipless baskets have greatly contributed to decreasing this risk. The key point to avoid any ureteral injury, and mainly avulsion, during stone manipulation with baskets, is to follow the basket and the entrapped stone all the way down the ureter by putting the ureteroscope just distal to the basket. In any case that force is needed during the extraction, the stone should be released under vision and stone disintegration should be performed until the creation of small enough fragments for safe removal. In the case that a ureteral stricture is the cause for stone extraction failure, a double J stent may be inserted for 2 weeks to assist in passive ureteral dilatation.

A common complication during ureteroscopy that may lead to avulsion is entrapment of the ureteral stonebasket. Forceful removal of the basket may tear the ureteral wall and cause partial or complete avulsion. To manage this complication and to avoid ureteral damage, the ureteroscope should be removed, after cutting the proximal part of the basket in order the ureteroscope to be removed from the working channel. In case that a ureteroscope with two working channels is used, this step can be omitted. The ureteroscope can then re-enter the ureter alongside the basket and the laser is used to break the basket wires. Following stone release, the basket is removed and lithotripsy may be continued. Alternatively, stone can be disintegrated within the basket and as soon as the fragments are small enough, basket can be removed with the fragments.

Ureteral avulsion rates are generally low in many large series. Geavlete et al. reported a 0.7 % rate (19 cases) of entrapped baskets in a series of 2,735 cases [2]. Eighteen cases were treated endoscopically while the rest one was treated with open ureterolithotomy and basket extraction. More recently, Tepeler et al. reported that stone avulsion was observed in 0.16 % of 1,208 patients treated with ureteroscopic lithotripsy for ureteral stones [1].

Most ureteral avulsions are recognized intraoperatively and can be managed at the same time. In the rare case that this is not identified during the procedure, early signs are flank pain and fever. Diagnosis can be confirmed with CT urography or antegrade ureterography by contrast extravasation and lack of contrast in the proximal ureter. Open or laparoscopic anastomosis of the ureter is the management of choice. The exact technique depends on the level and degree of avulsion. In case that a delayed correction is chosen, a percutaneous nephrostomy should be inserted for urine drainage.

Take Home Points

- Ureteroscopy is a relatively safe procedure for the treatment of ureteral stones with a low incidence of complications.
- Proper technique and experience are the mainstays for a safe procedure
- Most ureteral complications can be managed by a ureteral stent insertion.
- Forceful maneuvers during stone extraction should be avoided in order to decrease the risk of ureteral avulsion.
- Performing endoscopic maneuvers under direct visualization can minimize the incidence of major complications (ureteral perforation, significant ureteral bleeding, ureteral avulsion).

References

1. Tepeler A, Resorlu B, Sahin T, Sarikaya S, Bayindir M, Oguz U, et al. Categorization of intra-operative ureteroscopy complications using modified Satava classification system. World J Urol. 2014;32:131–6.
2. Geavlete P, Georgescu D, Niţă G, Mirciulescu V, Cauni V. Complications of 2735 retrograde semirigid ureteroscopy procedures: a single-center experience. J Endourol. 2006;20:179–85.
3. Watterson JD, Girvan AR, Cook AJ, Beiko DT, Nott L, Auge BK, et al. Safety and efficacy of holmium: YAG laser lithotripsy in patients with bleeding diatheses. J Urol. 2002;168:442–5.
4. Toepfer NJ, Baylor K, Henry Y, Simmons J, Berger PB. The effect of antiplatelet and anticoagulant therapy on the clinical outcome of patients undergoing ureteroscopy. Urology. 2013;82:773–9.
5. Abdel-Razzak O, Bagley DH. The 6.9F semirigid ureteroscope in clinical use. Urology. 1993;41:45–8.
6. Sofer M, Watterson JD, Wollin TA, Nott L, Razvi H, Denstedt JD. Holmium:YAG laser lithotripsy for upper urinary tract calculi in 598 patients. J Urol. 2002;167:31–4.
7. Başar H, Ohta N, Kageyama S, Suzuki K, Kawabe K. Treatment of ureteral and renal stones by electrohydraulic lithotripsy. Int Urol Nephrol. 1997;29:275–80.
8. Butler MR, Power RE, Thornhill JA, Ahmad I, McLornan I, McDermott T, et al. An audit of 2273 ureteroscopies–a focus on intra-operative complications to justify proactive management of ureteric calculi. Surgeon. 2004;2:42–6.
9. Francesca F, Scattoni V, Nava L, Pompa P, Grasso M, Rigatti P. Failures and complications of transurethral ureteroscopy in 297 cases: conventional rigid instruments vs. small caliber semirigid ureteroscopes. Eur Urol. 1995;28:112–5.
10. Al-Awadi K, Kehinde EO, Al-Hunayan A, Al-Khayat A. Iatrogenic ureteric injuries: incidence, aetiological factors and the effect of early management on subsequent outcome. Int Urol Nephrol. 2005;37:235–41.
11. Grasso M, Bagley D. Small diameter, actively deflectable, flexible ureteropyeloscopy. J Urol. 1998;160:1648–53.
12. Abdel-Razzak OM, Bagley DH. Clinical experience with flexible ureteropyeloscopy. J Urol. 1992;148:1788–92.
13. Bilen CY, Mahalati K, Sahin A, Tekin I, Ozen H, Remzi D. Ureteroscopic management of lower ureteral stones: two years' experience. Int Urol Nephrol. 1997;29:301–6.

14. Sözen S, Küpeli B, Tunc L, Senocak C, Alkibay T, Karaoğlan U, et al. Management of ureteral stones with pneumatic lithotripsy: report of 500 patients. J Endourol. 2003;17:721–4.
15. Aghamir SK, Mohseni MG, Ardestani A. Treatment of ureteral calculi with ballistic lithotripsy. J Endourol. 2003;17:887–90.
16. Hofbauer J, Höbarth K, Marberger M. Electrohydraulic versus pneumatic disintegration in the treatment of ureteral stones: a randomized, prospective trial. J Urol. 1995;153:623–5.
17. Sun Y, Wang L, Liao G, Xu C, Gao X, Yang Q, et al. Pneumatic lithotripsy versus laser lithotripsy in the endoscopic treatment of ureteral calculi. J Endourol. 2001;15:587–90.

Chapter 16
Future Directions

Sutchin R. Patel and Stephen Y. Nakada

As we have seen from the history of the treatment of ureteral stones to our current management, many of our advances have occurred because we have truly "stood on the shoulder of giants." We have progressed from cutting for stone to the era of endourology due to advances in numerous fields including radiology, the development of SWL, improvements in optics and the ureteroscope and the utilization of the laser for lithotripsy. In this chapter we will look to the future and hope to scour the horizon for the technological advances that will continue to revolutionize our field.

Ferromagnetic Extraction of Stone Fragments

The novel concept of removing stone fragments with a magnetic tool was first described by Tracy et al. in 2010 [1]. In order for stone fragments to be extracted with a magnet, the calcium based stones had to first be coated with solution that had a polymer that allowed binding to the stone attached to 1 μm microparticles with an iron oxide core (Invitrogen, Carlsberg USA). Tracy et al. then placed the coated stone fragments in a bladder model and found a 53 % reduction time in the extraction of the stone fragments compared to a 2.4Fr tipless nitinol basket [1].

Evaluation of the performance envelope for stone capture found that target capture was effective in the low, single digit millimeter distance range favoring smaller stones up to 3 mm in diameter [2]. An in vitro comparison of the magnetic tool with a conventional nitinol basket for ureteroscopic stone retrieval in a bench top simulator found that the magnetic tool improved the efficiency of retrieving stone particles

S.R. Patel, MD (✉) • S.Y. Nakada, MD
Department of Urology, University of Wisconsin School of Medicine and Public Health, Madison, WI, USA
e-mail: sutchin_patel@yahoo.com; nakada@urology.wisc.edu

S.R. Patel, S.Y. Nakada (eds.), *Ureteral Stone Management: A Practical Approach*, DOI 10.1007/978-3-319-08792-4_16

rendered paramagnetic that were less than 2 mm but showed no advantage for larger fragments [3]. The toxicity of the iron oxide microparticles was evaluated in a murine model [4]. The microparticles were not found to cross intact urothelial membranes and when introduced systemically, they led to minimal inflammatory changes in the lung and liver, thus additional longer term studies will be required to further assess toxicity.

Though the ferromagnetic extraction of stone fragment model was mainly devised in the case of fragment extraction during ureteroscopy and laser lithotripsy for renal stones or via PCNL it may also be applicable for ureteral stones [5]. The use of a magnetic tool versus a nitinol basket would: (1) allow easier extraction of smaller stone fragments, which can be difficult to basket extract (2) result in less passes in the ureter compared to the use of the basket for stone extraction thus leading to less ureteral trauma and perhaps even negating the risks of ureteral avulsion (3) aid in the extraction of stone fragments when there is poor visualization from bleeding. After this promising technique is further developed, human clinical trials will be required to evaluate its efficacy and applicability compared to stone basket extraction.

Robotic Flexible Ureteroscopy

The flexible Sensai® robotic catheter system (Hansen Medical System, Mountain View, CA) has been applied for robotic flexible ureteroscopy [6]. The system is based on a remote master-slave system that consists of: (1) a surgeon console, including the master input device (MID) (2) remote catheter manipulator (3) the flexible catheter system (4) an electronics rack which contains all the video and computer hardware. The MID has a 3-dimensional joystick that the surgeon uses to manipulate the catheter tip. The display monitor shows endoscopic visualization, real-time fluoroscopic views and a catheter animation on the LCD display that gives the surgeon the location and orientation of the ureteroscope tip in the collecting system. The remote element consists of the remote catheter manipulator which is an arm that attaches to the operating table on which the steerable catheter sheath and guide catheter are attached [6]. The robotic system is built to treat renal stones as the flexible ureteroscope is fixed to and guided by the inner catheter (10–12Fr) which is placed through an outer catheter sheath (12–14Fr) which stabilizes the inner catheter at the level of the ureteropelvic junction. The maximum deflection of the flexible catheter system is 270°.

Desai et al. performed the preliminary animal studies of the flexible ureteroscope robotic system in the swine model and demonstrated ureteroscopy with holmium laser lithotripsy of 4 mm human stones that had been placed in the kidneys [7]. Balloon dilation of the ureter was required in 2/10 ureters to accommodate the robotic catheter system. The early animal studies allowed for further changes to the robotic system including decreasing the diameter of the robotic ureteroscope to improve drainage of the irrigant fluid.

The first clinical study using the flexible ureteroscopy robotic system was performed in 2011 when 18 patients with renal calculi were treated [8]. All patients did have pre-existing ureteral stents in place 2 weeks prior to the procedure. Flexible robotic ureteroscopy with laser lithotripsy was performed successfully in all 18 patients. The mean operative time was 91 min, the mean stone size was 11.8 mm, mean robotic docking time was 7.3 min and total robot time including docking time was 41.4 min. No intraoperative complications were observed and there was no evidence of renal perforation as confirmed by contrast injection at the end of each case. Complete stone free status was achieved in ten patients (56 %) at 2 months based on CT-imaging and 15 patients (89 %) at 3 months based on intravenous pyelogram. One patient required an auxiliary procedure for clearance of symptomatic residual stone debris. There was no evidence of ureteral stricture on follow-up at 3 months.

The development of flexible robotic technology was the potential to have numerous applications across many other surgical specialties [9]. One benefit of flexible robotic ureteroscopy is the application of motion scaling with fine scaling advantageous in the targeting and treatment of small stone fragments. By using a remote surgical system with a master-slave system, the surgeon is no longer at the bedside and thus is not exposed to any radiation via fluoroscopy. One of the disadvantages of the robotic system is the lack of haptic feedback which plays a significant role in current flexible ureteroscopy and which may prevent inadvertent tissue injury.

The preliminary results from the flexible robotic ureteroscopy system appear to be promising. Further technological improvements followed by trials comparing manual ureteroscopy to the robotic system will be needed to evaluate the benefits and economic feasibility of the flexible robotic ureteroscopy system.

Ultrasonic Propusion of Urolithiasis

The use of focused ultrasonic propulsion to move renal calculi in the collecting system is a novel technique to help pass renal calculi and potentially relieve an obstructing ureteral stone by moving it into the renal pelvis [10]. Harper et al. showed that focused ultrasonic propulsion was used to successfully relocate 17 of 26 stones (65 %) in a mean procedure time of 14 min utilizing a mean of 23 ultrasound bursts [10]. Successful stone relocation was defined as stone movement from the calyx to the renal pelvis, ureteropelvic junction or proximal ureter. Transcutaneous ultrasonic propulsion was performed using an HDI C5-2 imaging transducer (ATL/ Phillips, Bothell, WA) and the Verasconics® diagnostic ultrasound platform.

The acoustic pressure and energy for this technique are lower than those used currently for SWL so it was hypothesized that the technique would lead to minimal renal injury. Connors et al. showed that focused ultrasonic propulsion produced no detectable morphological injury to renal parenchyma in a porcine model when using clinical treatment parameters, but produced injury comparable in size to SWL when using excessive treatment parameters [11].

As focused ultrasonic propulsion of renal calculi undergoes clinical testing it may be useful in a number of scenarios [12]. It may be used as an adjunct to primary medical expulsive therapy for smaller stones or after lithotripsy to clear residual fragments. It may have a role in the management of acute renal colic due to an obstructing UPJ stone by pushing the stone back into a nonobstructing location. It may also have an adjunctive role in an intraoperative setting allowing for the repositioning of stones during ureteroscopy or percutaneous nephrolithotomy to allow for easier treatment or stone extraction.

Burst Wave Lithotripsy

Burst wave lithotripsy is an experimental method to noninvasively fragment urolithiasis using focused bursts of ultrasound [13]. Burst wave lithotripsy utilizes focused sinusoidal ultrasound bursts rather than shock waves to disintegrate stones into small fragments. Similar to SWL, BWL's mechanism for fragmentation of stone is based on a combination of pressure waves inside the stone due to the incident sound field and cavitation effects at the stone surface. While SWL is broadband in nature which leads to a wide distribution of stone fragments, BWL has a narrowband nature leading to control of fragment size. Because the cavitation bubble growth is significantly less than SWL, it therefore allows for energy to be delivered at a higher rate and allows potentially for less injury. BWL appears to be a promising new technology that may be utilized for stone fragmentation. However further studies will be needed to evaluate its effectiveness and potential tissue injury prior to clinical trials.

Stone Prevention and Quality of Life

Though our text has focused on the treatment of ureteral stones, stone prevention via medical management and dietary recommendations has become increasingly important as the incidence of stone disease has risen. The recent publication of the AUA Guidelines on the Medical Management of Kidney Stones has codified and organized our approach to preventing urolithiasis, illustrated the available data to support the recommendations by the panel and highlighted areas where further research and studies need to be performed [14]. When measuring the effectiveness of treatment for ureteral stones we have primarily focused on clinical endpoints such as stone free rates or complication rates. The assessment of patient health related quality of life for stone formers is important in that it is an outcome that is relevant to the patient, not solely the disease process, and may affect decisions made regarding medical and surgical management. The Wisconsin Stone QOL, a disease specific assessment tool for stone formers, helps to capture the patient reported aspects of urolithiasis related symptoms [15]. Future assessment of health related quality of life for stone formers at various points before, during and after their treatment will aid us in identifying how to better treat our patients.

Take Home Points

- The development of ferromagnetic extraction of stone fragments may lead to higher stone free rates and less passages up the ureter for stone extraction in the future.
- The fine scaling of flexible robotic ureteroscopy may help in the treatment of smaller stone fragments and the flexible robot may also have applications across multiple surgical disciplines.
- Focused ultrasonic propulsion of urolithiasis may be useful in many clinical scenarios including aid in the passage of small stone fragments, pushing an obstructing UPJ stone back into the renal pelvis during an episode of renal colic or as an adjunct to ureteroscopy or PCNL to aid in stone treatment and extraction.
- Burst wave lithotripsy is a promising experimental method to noninvasively fragment urolithiasis using focused sinusoidal ultrasound bursts.
- Health related quality of life assessment may have equivalent value to stone free rates as a measurable patient outcome in the future.

References

1. Tracy CR, McLeroy SL, Best SL, Gnade BE, Pearle MS, Cadeddu JA. Rendering stone fragments paramagnetic with iron-oxide microparticles improves the efficiency and effectiveness of endoscopic stone fragment retrieval. Urology. 2010;76(5):1266.e10–4.
2. Fernandez R, Tan YK, Kaberle W, Best SL, Olweny EO, Pearle MS, Gnade BE, McElroy SL, Cadeddu JA. Determining a performance envelope for capture of kidney stones functionalized with superparamagnetic microparticles. J Endourol. 2012;26(9):1227–30.
3. Tan YK, McLeroy SL, Faddegon S, Olweny E, Fernandez R, Beardsley H, Gnade B, Park S, Pearle MS, Cadeddu JA. In vitro comparison of prototype magnetic tool with conventional nitinol basket for ureteroscopic retrieval of stone fragments rendered paramagnetic with iron oxide microparticles. J Urol. 2012;188(2):648–52.
4. Tan YK, Best SL, Donnelly C, Olweny E, Kapur P, Mir SA, Gnade B, McLEroy S, Pearle MS, Cadeddu JA. Novel iron oxide microparticles used to render stone fragments paramagnetic: assessment of toxicity in a murine model. J Urol. 2012;188(5):1972–7.
5. Tan YK, Pearle MS, Cadeddu JA. Rendering stone fragments paramagnetic with iron-oxide microparticles to improve the efficiency of endoscopic stone fragment retrieval. Curr Opin Urol. 2012;22(2):144–7.
6. Lee DJ, Desai MM. Robotics. In: Monga M, editor. Ureteroscopy: indications & technique. New York: Springer Science & Business Media; 2013. Chapter 38.
7. Desai MM, Aron M, Gill IS, Pascal-Haber G, Ukimura O, Kaouk JH, Stahler G, Barbagli F, Carlson C, Moll F. Flexible robotic retrograde renoscopy: description of novel robotic device and preliminary laboratory experience. Urology. 2008;72(1):42–6.
8. Desai MM, Grover R, Aron M, Ganpule A, Joshi SS, Desai MR, Gill IS. Robotic flexible ureteroscopy for renal calculi: initial clinical experience. J Urol. 2011;186(2):563–8.
9. Canes D, Lehman AC, Farritor SM, Oleynikov D, Desai MM. The future of NOTES instrumentation: flexible robotics and in vivo minirobots. J Endourol. 2009;23(5):787–92.
10. Harper JD, Sorensen MD, Cunitz BW, Wang YN, Simon JC, Starr F, Paun M, Dunmire B, Liggitt HD, Evan AP, McAteer JA, His RS, Bailey MR. Focused ultrasound to expel calculi from the kidney: safety and efficacy of a clinical prototype device. J Urol. 2013;190(3):1090–5.

11. Connors BA, Evan AP, Blomgren PM, Hsi RS, Harper JD, Sorensen MD, Wang YN, Simon JC, Paun M, Starr F, Cunitz BW, Bailey MR, Lingeman JE. Comparison of tissue injury from focused ultrasonic propulsion of kidney stones versus shock wave lithotripsy. J Urol. 2014;191(1):235–41.
12. Sorensen MD, Bailey MR, Hsi RS, Cunitz BW, Simon JC, Wang YN, Dunmire BL, Paun M, Starr F, Lu W, Evan AP, Harper JD. Focused ultrasonic propulsion of kidney stones: review and update of preclinical technology. J Endourol. 2013;27(10):1183–6.
13. Maxwell A, Kreider W, Cuntz B, Wang Y, His R, Lee F, Harper J, Bailey M. Evaluation of stone comminution and tissue injury in vivo using a novel method of lithotripsy without shock waves. J Urol. 2014;191(4):e946.
14. Pearle MS, Goldfarb DS, Assimos DG, Curhan G, Denu-Ciocca CJ, Matlaga BR, Monga M, Penniston KL, Preminger GM, Turk TM, White JR. Medical management of kidney stones: AUA guideline. J Urol. 2014;19:316–24. Epub May 20, 2014.
15. Penniston KL, Nakada SY. Development of an instrument to assess the health related quality of life of kidney stone formers. J Urol. 2013;189:921–30.

Index

S.R. Patel, S.Y. Nakada (eds.), *Ureteral Stone Management: A Practical Approach*, DOI 10.1007/978-3-319-08792-4

V

MIX
Papier aus verantwortungsvollen Quellen
Paper from responsible sources
FSC® C105338

If you have any concerns about our products,
you can contact us on
ProductSafety@springernature.com

In case Publisher is established outside the EU,
the EU authorized representative is:
Springer Nature Customer Service Center GmbH
Europaplatz 3, 69115 Heidelberg, Germany

Printed by Libri Plureos GmbH
in Hamburg, Germany